THE
SIX–WEEK
FAT-TO-MUSCLE
MAKEOVER

■ ELLINGTON DARDEN, PH.D. ■

THE

SIX–WEEK

FAT-TO-MUSCLE

MAKEOVER

A PERIGEE BOOK

NOTICE: Reduced diet and strenuous exercise may not be advisable for persons with certain medical conditions. It is highly recommended that the reader consult with a physician before beginning the program presented in this book or any other diet and exercise program. Responsibility for any adverse effects or unforeseen consequences resulting from the use of any information contained herein is expressly disclaimed, and rests solely with the reader.

Perigee Books
are published by
The Putnam Publishing Group
200 Madison Avenue
New York, NY 10016

First Perigee Edition 1990
Copyright © 1988 by Ellington Darden, Ph.D.

Library of Congress Cataloging-in-Publication Data

Darden, Ellington, date.
   The six-week fat-to-muscle makeover / by Ellington Darden.
      p.   cm.
   1. Reducing exercises.   2. Weight lifting.   3. Exercise for women.
4. Reducing diets.   I. Darden, Ellington, date.   II. Title.
RA781.6.D38   1989   89-8597 CIP
646.7'5—dc20
ISBN 0-399-51562-3

Cover design copyright © 1988 by Andrew M. Newman
Front cover photograph by Dan Howard
Front cover model: Connie May, age 25, who lost 15 pounds in six weeks

Book design and composition by The Sarabande Press
Printed in the United States of America

ACKNOWLEDGMENTS

To Terry Duschinski, my most grateful appreciation for your assistance in writing this book.

Thank you, Timothy Tew, for your great job on the exercise photography in Chapters 11 and 12, as well as the portrait photography in Chapter 1.

Thanks to Kevin Berry for the hair and face makeovers in Chapter 1.

Thank you, Ken Hutchins, for your precise work on the before-and-after photography for this project.

Appreciation to Bob Sikora for your skill in challenging women to get maximum results out of their Nautilus exercise.

Thanks to Brenda Hutchins for your menu and recipe planning.

And special thanks to Pat Schroeder of the Absolute Casting Agency, Tampa, Florida; Joe Cirulli of the Gainesville Health and Fitness Center, Gainesville, Florida; Jim Randall of the Lincoln Fitness Center, Orlando, Florida; Terry Duschinski of Firm & Fit, DeLand, Florida; and all the Florida women who participated in the research for this book.

CONTENTS

PART I

▪UNDERSTANDING▪

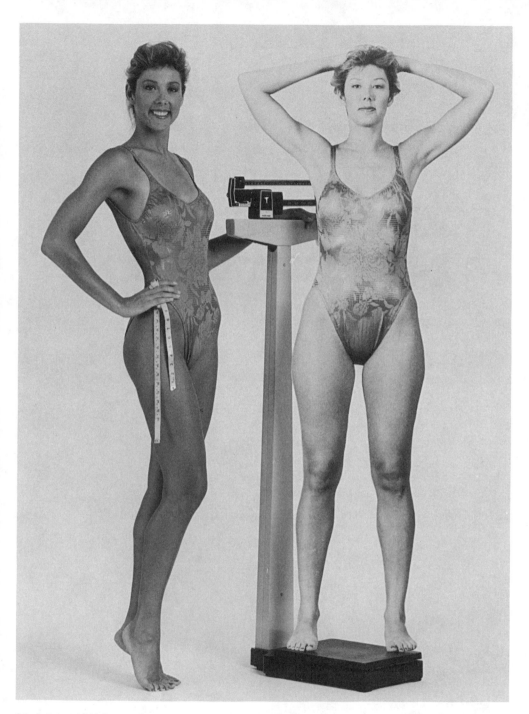

Madelaine Wildman, seen here standing next to a life-size picture of the way her body looked prior to the start of the program, is positive proof of the effectiveness of the Six-Week Fat-to-Muscle Makeover. Madelaine lost 18¼ pounds of fat and added 4½ pounds of muscle—in only six weeks!

▪FAT-TO-MUSCLE MAKEOVERS▪

Faces, chests, shoulders, waists, hips, thighs, and legs.

BODIES! These are what we concentrate on when we meet people.

First impressions, especially when women are involved, go back to the king of the senses: the eyes. What we see—more than what we hear, feel, taste, or smell—is what we tend to remember.

Sigmund Freud said it best more than eighty years ago: "anatomy is destiny."

Sure, clothes make the man (and woman), as the old saying goes. But what lends form to the clothes? Only one thing—the body.

The body that is in this year at the beach, on a picnic, on a cruise, on the ski slopes, on the dance floor, and at the fitness center is certainly not fat and flabby. It's lean, strong, firm, and shapely.

A lean, strong, firm, and shapely body in the past has been primarily a result of good genetics. Usually, a well-built woman was born that way. Maybe she did a little dieting and exercising, but most of her attractive figure was in spite of her practices, not because of them. Much of her dieting and exercising actually could have been detrimental because of the abundance of misinformation and dangerous products on the market.

Were a genetically gifted woman to involve herself in proper diet and proper exercise, in a matter of weeks she would attain results that would exceed her expectations. Genetics plus science would produce an absolutely stunning body.

The more typical woman also falls short of her body's potential because she does not understand and apply scientific principles to her diet and exercise programs.

A 1986 survey by the advertising agency D'Arcy, Masius, Benton & Bowles, Inc., reveals that, even though more American women than ever before are actively trying to get fit, 88 percent of them still want to weigh less. Primarily, they want to lose pounds and inches from their waists, hips, and thighs.

Look no more. Now there's a program that actually does what it claims to do. It makes over the figure by changing the muscle-to-fat ratio. It reshapes the body by building muscle and reducing fat. And it works for almost any woman.

THE MAKEOVER PROJECT

In 1985 I supervised the dieting and exercising of sixty-five women and thirty-three men in a ten-week program at the Gainesville Health and Fitness Center in Gainesville, Florida. The average woman in this program lost 18¾ pounds of fat and the average man lost 30 pounds. The fat-loss results were so significant that a 416-

page book, *The Nautilus Diet* (Boston: Little, Brown, 1987), was published to explain the program. Since the publication of *The Nautilus Diet,* many women have asked me if I had an abbreviated program for those who needed to lose less weight than 18 pounds — say only 5, 10, or 15 pounds.

With that objective in mind, I organized a six-week diet and exercise program. To test my new plan, I contacted a friend in Tampa, Florida, who owned a modeling agency. Within several days she recruited twenty-nine women who needed to lose between 5 and 15 pounds.

In the spring of 1986 these women were placed on a specific descending-calorie diet combined with three-times-a-week Nautilus exercise. The overall results were gratifying. In six weeks, most of the women exceeded their body-shaping goals.

The program, in my estimation, still needed simplification and further testing. In the fall of 1986, I went to Gainesville, Florida, and organized another group of twenty-one women. With this group I introduced a new style of Nautilus training, called *super slow.* This style of training involves a very slow repetition — 10 seconds on the lifting phase, and 4 seconds lowering.

The overall achievements of this super-slow group proved to be the best I had experienced in my many years of working with overfat and out-of-shape women.

To make sure that the results of the super-slow group were not a fluke, in 1987 I supervised a third and fourth group of women in Orlando through the same six-week program.

The Orlando groups' achievements reinforced the evidence that slow, deliberate exercise movements are better than faster movements for overall body shaping and fat loss. Since then I've tested the same program several more times, with small groups of women in DeLand, Florida, and in Orlando. I've examined the effects of this program on average overfat women, grossly overfat women, slim models who were not overfat but undermuscled, athletes, and women who did not have access to Nautilus equipment. The results were dramatic in almost every case.

WHAT TO EXPECT

In all, ninety women took part in the research for this book. Before-and-after measurements for the ninety women show that, in six weeks, each lost an average of:

- 12½ pounds of fat
- 2½ inches off the waist
- 1⅝ inches off the hips
- 1¼ inches off each thigh

These same women added an average of 3⅞ pounds of figure-shaping muscle each to their bodies. The above averages provide realistic expectations for most women who are motivated to follow the week-by-week course of action.

In this Fat-to-Muscle Makeover, a picture is worth a thousand measurements. That's why the rest of this chapter shares with you the real-life pictures, as well as the measurements and stories, of some of the women who went through the program.

The makeover effect is awesome.

SENSATIONAL SYBIL

Competitive bodybuilding was once central to Sybil King's existence. She trained compulsively, working out hour upon hour in the gym trying to get just a little more burn in the muscle, leading to just a little more bulge.

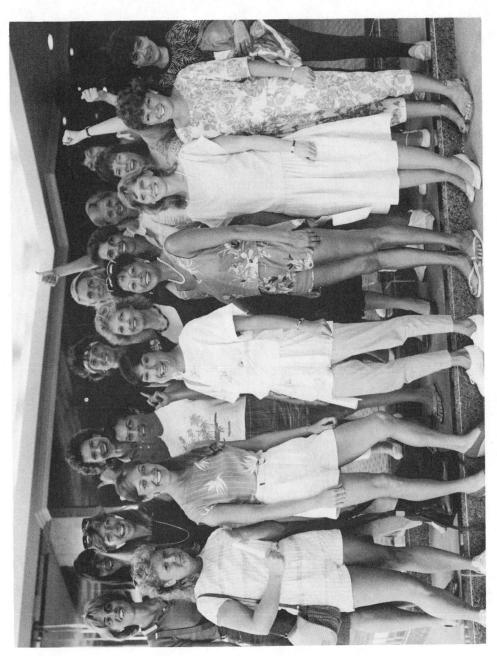

This photo shows some of the women who completed the Fat-to-Muscle Makeover in Tampa, Florida.

"I did it just to see if I could do it, but then I would never get into a contest," Sybil admitted.

"I would prepare; I would get ripped (bodybuilding term for extreme leanness), but then I would flake out."

While her feminine physique is very attractive, Sybil lacks the extraordinary genetic muscle-building makeup necessary for top-flight women's bodybuilding.

By age 27 she had exchanged her concern for getting ripped for the concerns of a wife and mother. But something had escaped that she had never wanted to lose. Stress built up. Finally Sybil realized that her physical condition was a bummer. She neither looked nor felt the way she once did, the way she wanted.

"I kept using the excuse that I'd just had a baby, but my baby was almost a year old," she said.

She was ready for a Fat-to-Muscle Makeover.

As part of the research group at the Lincoln Fitness Center in suburban Orlando, Sybil dropped 14½ pounds of fat, lowering her body fat from 28.2 percent to 19.6 percent. Her waistline was the biggest beneficiary, showing a 3-inch reduction.

But the changes in Sybil's anatomy can't match the psychological catharsis she underwent.

"I now handle stress much better both at work and at home," said Sybil, an administrative assistant at a computer company. "Working out keeps me from becoming irritable. It makes me more productive at business and happier at home."

Comparing her Six-Week Fat-to-Muscle Makeover conditioning program to the rigors of bodybuilding, Sybil explained:

"I'm happy where I am at now as a housewife, mother, and professional person. I'm happier with my body now than I ever was then. I'm healthy, I think I have a good-looking body, and I feel positive about myself."

SYBIL KING, AGE 27

"THIS DIET AND EXERCISE PROGRAM LIFTED MY SELF-ESTEEM FROM A LOW LEVEL TO THE HIGHEST IT HAS EVER BEEN."

Lost 14½ pounds of fat and trimmed 3 inches off her waist, 1⅞ inches off her hips, 2½ inches off her thighs in *six* weeks!

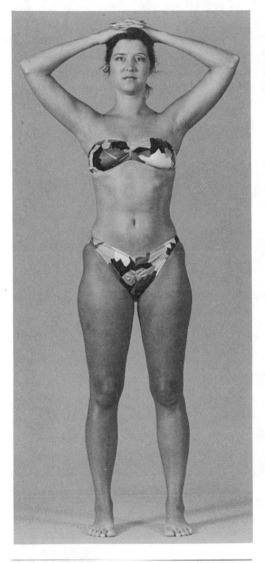 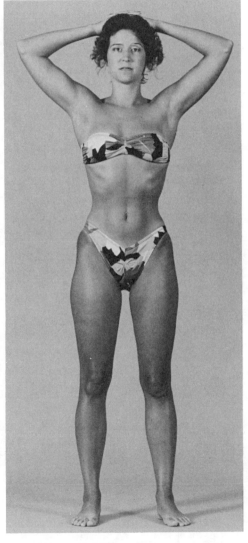

BEFORE
Six-Week Fat-to-Muscle Makeover.

AFTER
Six-Week Fat-to-Muscle Makeover.

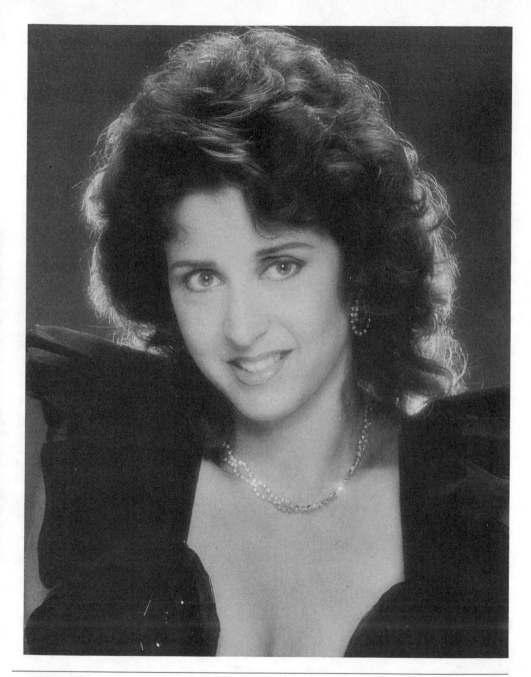

"WHEN I LOOK ATTRACTIVE, I FEEL GOOD ABOUT MYSELF. THIS FEELING TRANSFERS DIRECTLY TO MY HUSBAND AND CHILD."
—SYBIL KING

MADELAINE'S MAKEOVER

Madelaine Wildman used to speak enviously when explaining that she is from a family of "incredibly beautiful, thin women."

Her mother was a top cover girl with the renowned Eileen Ford Modeling Agency in New York City. Her sister is an actress in Hollywood. Her cousin is a high-fashion model working in New York City and Miami.

Madelaine, age 28, never felt quite up to par with those she shared family dinner with.

But she was trying. For ten years Madelaine had belonged to various fitness clubs. She was in search of a personal trainer when the Fat-to-Muscle Makeover research project at the Lincoln Fitness Center caught her attention.

Her fat-loss performance was tops in the group of twenty-eight women. "I'm on cloud nine," Madelaine rejoiced in an interview after the program's completion.

She trimmed 3 inches off each thigh—6 inches total—en route to an 18¼-pound fat-loss performance. Her waist also shrunk by 3 inches, and her hips lost 2⅜ inches.

"I worked harder at this program than anything I'd ever done in my life, and I got results I never dreamed possible," said Madelaine, who is a telecommunications manager.

"The response of my friends has been great. My female friends are both proud and envious—especially when I put on a pair of my friend Karen's jeans. She's an instructor at a health club and she's very thin.

"My male friends," Madelaine continued, "can't believe the changes. They tell me not to lose any more weight—I never thought I'd hear anyone say that! My ex-boyfriend is even calling me again."

Madelaine slipped into a bathing suit after the last of her six weeks

MADELAINE WILDMAN, AGE 28

"MY NEW BODY HAS GIVEN ME GREAT CONFIDENCE IN BOTH MY BUSINESS AND PERSONAL LIFE."

Lost 18¼ pounds of fat and trimmed 3 inches off her waist, 2⅜ inches off her hips, 6 inches off her thighs in *six* weeks!

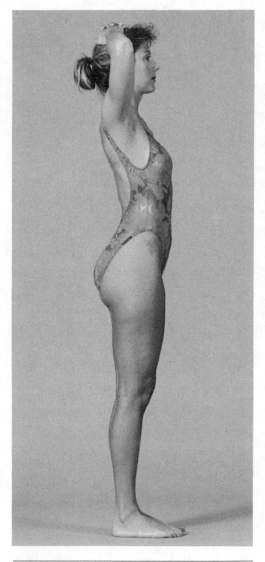

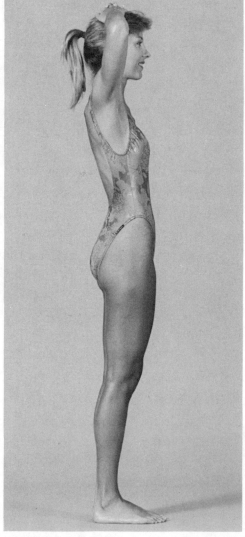

BEFORE
Six-Week Fat-to-Muscle Makeover.

AFTER
Six-Week Fat-to-Muscle Makeover.

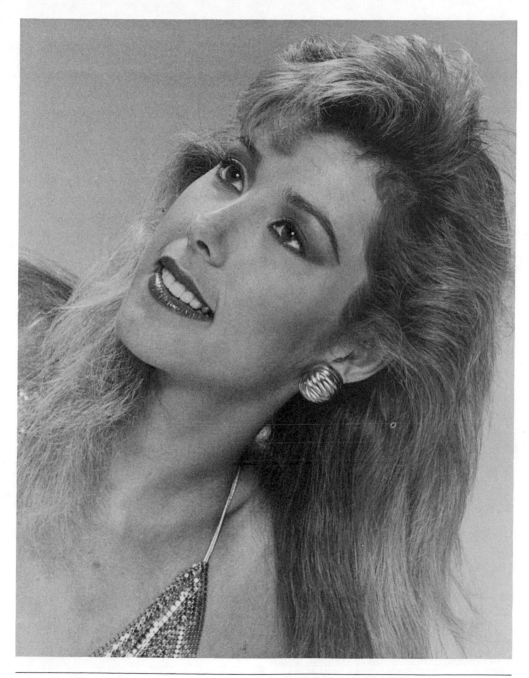

"I NOW REALIZE THAT LARGER, STRONGER MUSCLES ARE MY BEST ALLY AGAINST THE AGING PROCESS."
—MADELAINE WILDMAN

of workouts and had her instructor snap a few posing shots. She later showed the photos to an upstairs neighbor at her condominium complex, who insisted on taking the photos to her husband.

"A few minutes later," chuckled Madelaine, "my friend's husband called and said, 'I'm throwing my wife out—I just saw your pictures. In fact, you should see her flying by your window any second now!'"

The exhilarating experience, Madelaine indicates, will propel her to new heights.

"Through the Six-Week Fat-to-Muscle Makeover, I have dramatically changed my complete self-image," she said. "I feel I can achieve anything if I set my mind to it."

Due to excess pounds, most of which she picked up while in college, Madelaine thought she could never be in the league of her mother, sister, and cousin.

"I was always on the sidelines cheering them on," she said.

Not anymore.

LYSA SCULPTURES SHAPELIER FIGURE

Nineteen-year-old Lysa Parker is far from average. You wouldn't think that you could improve upon her lean, shapely figure. She entered the Fat-to-Muscle Makeover with only 15.5 percent body fat. Why would she even bother?

As a part-time professional model, her every curve, sag, and pouch is scrutinized. The competition for modeling assignments is fierce.

The Makeover program added weight to Lysa's 5-foot-6¼-inch frame. It also added inches in every area except one.

Lysa Parker's results exemplify the figure-shaping impact of added muscle.

Her scale weight rose by 1¼ pounds; however, her body-fat

LYSA PARKER, AGE 19

"I NEVER KNEW HOW WEAK I LOOKED, ESPECIALLY FROM THE BACK. ADDING MUSCLE HELPED MY POSTURE AND IMPROVED MY ENTIRE FIGURE."

Added 4 pounds of muscle and *gained* 2¼ inches on her back and chest, ½ inch on her upper arms, and *trimmed* 1 inch off her waist in *six* weeks!

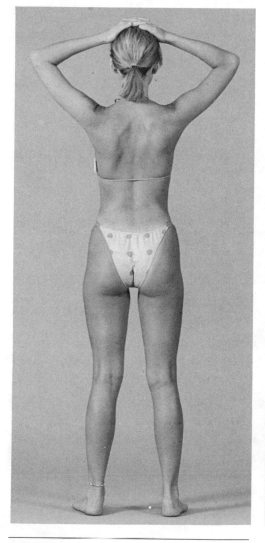

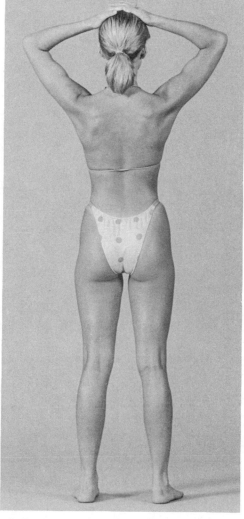

BEFORE
Six-Week Fat-to-Muscle Makeover.

AFTER
Six-Week Fat-to-Muscle Makeover.

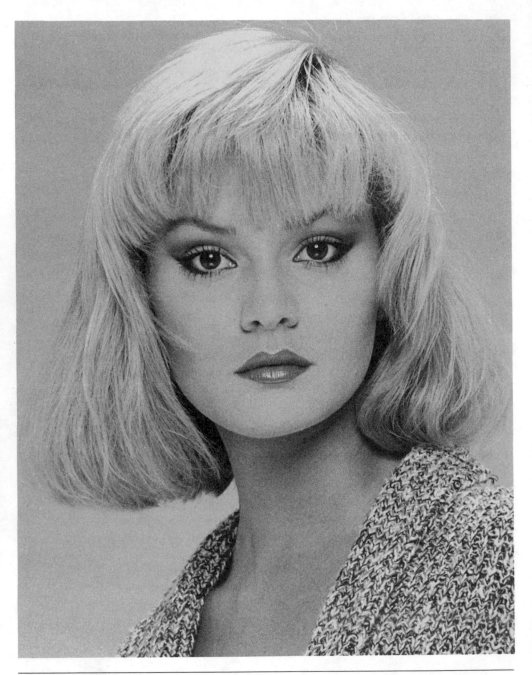

"THE MAKEOVER PROGRAM TAUGHT ME THE IMPORTANCE OF COMBINING A BALANCED DIET WITH INTENSE EXERCISE."
—LYSA PARKER

percentage decreased to 12.5 percent. She added fractions of inches to her arms, hips, and thighs—and did wonders for two vitally important areas of the feminine physique, especially in her line of work.

Lysa increased her chest measurement by 2¼ inches, and she trimmed an inch off her waist.

A close look at her before-and-after photos also reveals an improvement in her posture.

"My friends noticed the difference when we were at the beach," said Lysa. "Many people asked about my workouts and commented on how much more fit I look."

It is possible that Lysa's Makeover Diet was actually an increase in calories from her previous level. "That was a lot of food," she remarked.

But she added muscle that consumed the calories; enough to even burn fat from a body that carried very little fat to begin with.

"I can feel the difference," said Lysa. "It's evident in some of the clothes I wear. Certain kinds of fashions fit better. I have a better shape; I feel tighter—and much stronger.

"The productive career of a model is very short," Lysa went on to say. "This training program will sustain my career much longer than would otherwise be possible."

2

▪WHY THE FAT-TO-MUSCLE MAKEOVER WORKS▪

Over the last twenty-five years I've used, administered, and tested numerous diet and exercise plans. None of these plans, however, combats the overfat problems that women have as well as the Fat-to-Muscle Makeover program.

The Fat-to-Muscle Makeover program is effective in reshaping a woman's figure because it embraces four important concepts. It (1) decreases dietary calories, (2) increases exercise calories, (3) builds muscle mass, and (4) stresses maintenance and follow-up. Let's examine each of these factors.

DIETARY CALORIES

Decreasing dietary calories is the backbone of any successful fat-loss program. But unless the calories are decreased gradually—with the proper proportions of carbohydrates, fats, and proteins—most of the weight you lose will be from your muscles and blood, rather than your fat stores.

The initial phase of the Makeover Diet is composed of six weeks, or three two-week segments. You begin with 1,200 calories a day for the first two weeks. Each subsequent two-week segment decreases the total by 100 calories. Thus, during weeks 5 and 6, you are at the 1,000-calorie level. This is the lowest number of calories that you will consume, and you'll never remain at that level for longer than two weeks at a time.

Those who stay on the diet longer than six weeks raise their daily calories to 1,200 in the seventh week and repeat the gradual descent in three two-week segments for as long as necessary.

The proportions of carbohydrates, fats, and proteins remain constant throughout the daily menus:

- 50 percent carbohydrates
- 30 percent fats
- 20 percent proteins

All you have to do is follow the menus and recipes exactly as directed in Part II of this book.

EXERCISE CALORIES

As your dietary calories decrease slowly, the calories you burn from exercise do the opposite: they increase with each two-week segment.

TANYA PELTO, AGE 50

"I FEEL MUCH BETTER PHYSICALLY—AND MORE SURE OF MY-SELF. MY HUSBAND IS SO PROUD OF ME. HE STILL CALLS ME HIS BRIDE—NOW WITH A LITTLE BUTT."

Lost 18 pounds of fat and trimmed 3⅞ inches off her waist, 1⅜ inches off her hips, 4¾ inches off her thighs in *six* weeks!

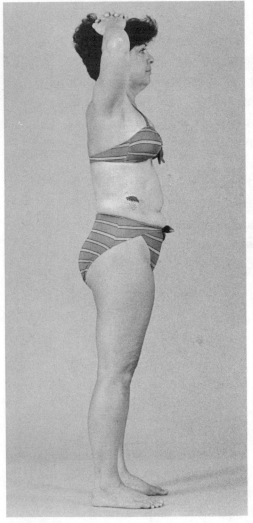

BEFORE
Six-Week Fat-to-Muscle Makeover.

AFTER
Six-Week Fat-to-Muscle Makeover.

Calories burned from exercise are dependent on the intensity and duration of the movement.

For the first two weeks, participants perform six basic exercises. They progress to eight exercises for the next two weeks, then ten for weeks 5 and 6.

Furthermore, as the duration of the exercise session increases, the resistance (weight) used—if proper intensity is employed—becomes progressively heavier and heavier. The calorie-burning potential of progressive-resistance exercise, especially that performed on Nautilus equipment, is second to none. It not only burns calories while you do the exercise, but it also burns calories while you're resting. Burning calories at rest is directly related to the amount of muscle on your body.

BUILDING MUSCLE MASS

Traditionally, there have been two ways to lose fat: decrease your dietary calories and increase your exercise calories. The Fat-to-Muscle Makeover program actively promotes a third way: it causes your body to use more calories in ways that do not involve exertion.

The primary way to cause your body to burn calories at rest is by building your muscles. Larger muscles, more than anything else that you have control over, need calories to function. Add 1 pound of muscle to your body and it automatically requires an additional 50 to 100 calories per day.

During my six-week studies in Florida the average woman added almost 4 pounds of muscle to her body. This extra muscle mass raised each participant's fat-burning metabolism. It also improved her physical appearance. And most important, building muscle increased her probability of keeping the lost fat off permanently.

The reduction in circumference inches, incidentally, is truly more dramatic than the numbers on the scale. In just six weeks you can easily drop three dress or pants sizes! Many women in Florida did.

"I have pants that look like a person moved out," said Karen Houck, after losing only 7 pounds of scale weight. Another Florida woman, Katie Timko lost 13 pounds of fat and termed the effect on her figure "amazing. It's amazing that you can do that in just six weeks."

Do not underestimate the importance of building muscle to lose fat. It works in a very dramatic fashion as you can see from the before-and-after photographs in this book.

MAINTENANCE AND FOLLOW-UP

Most people who lose significant amounts of fat gain it back within the first year. Such individuals are willing to restrict themselves for only a few months, and several months won't last a lifetime.

The key to keeping your lost fat off is your muscle-fat ratio. The Fat-to-Muscle Makeover program provides the necessary guidelines and follow-up you need to stabilize your muscle-fat ratio at the optimum level for the rest of your life.

"The program taught me how to be in control," said one of the successful Gainesville participants, "in control of my eating, exercising, and total life-style. I'll never be fat again!"

Being in control does not mean that you are restricted by what you can and cannot eat for the rest of your life. It means that you can now eat anything you want — in moderation and with certain short-range adjustments.

MARGARET LACROIX, AGE 38

"NOW I CAN WEAR THE CLOTHES I HAVE HAD HANGING IN MY CLOSET FOR TWO YEARS. EVERYONE SAYS I LOOK SO MUCH BETTER, AND I REALLY FEEL 100% BETTER."

Lost 22½ pounds of fat and trimmed 4⅝ inches off her waist, 2⅜ inches off her hips, 4¼ inches off her thighs in *six* weeks!

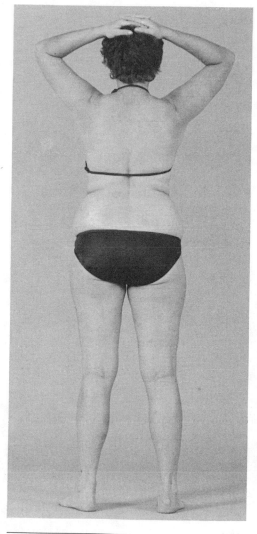

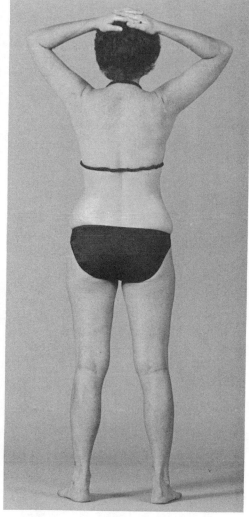

BEFORE
Six-Week Fat-to-Muscle Makeover.

AFTER
Six-Week Fat-to-Muscle Makeover.

ONE STEP AT A TIME

An understanding of the concepts presented in this chapter is the initial step in reshaping your body. The next chapter involves a discussion of your muscle-fat ratio.

3

▪MUSCLE-FAT RATIO ▪

If you find yourself afflicted with flabby thighs, saddlebag hips, or a protruding stomach, you want nothing more than to firm, tone, and sculpt a more attractive physique. I have found very few women who are totally satisfied with their figures. Size 14 women want to wear a size 8, and size 6 women want to wear a size 4.

Everybody wants to improve.

In this quest for firmness it's important to understand something far more important than scale weight.

Your primary concern should be your *muscle-to-fat ratio*. This is a comparison on the number of pounds of muscle on your body to pounds of fat.

BODY COMPOSITION OF THE AVERAGE WOMAN

Ten years ago the average woman in the United States was 28 years old, 5 feet, 4 inches tall, and weighed 135 pounds. Today she is 32 years old, still 5 feet, 4 inches tall, but weighs 143 pounds.

The exercise phenomenon in this country hasn't enabled the average woman to become leaner, but instead has left her 8 pounds heavier. Her body tissue is composed of:

- 12 percent bone
- 26 percent organs
- 36 percent muscle
- 26 percent fat

Of the four components only her muscle and fat are subject to significant modification through diet and exercise. Her muscle-fat ratio amounts to 1.38 pounds of muscle for each 1.0 pounds of fat. Such a ratio is far from ideal. The typical woman's body is overfat and flabby.

She needs less fat and more muscle. A realistic six-week goal is to lose 13 pounds of fat and gain 3 pounds of muscle. Doing so would reduce this average woman's weight from 143 to 133. It would also change her muscle-fat ratio from 1.38/1 to 2.25/1. In the process, her percentage of body fat would drop from 26 to 18. Especially striking would be her smaller waist and leaner thighs.

Many of the women who took part in the Fat-to-Muscle Makeover reduced their body fat to 18 percent or lower. I consider 16–18 percent to be ideal for most middle-aged women. I'll show you how to estimate your percentage of body fat later in this chapter.

For now, the main concept that you need to understand is that the quality of your figure is determined to a great extent, not by how much you weigh, but by your muscle-fat ratio.

IMPROVED BODY SHAPE

The primary determinant of the body's shape is its bones. But after the bones, the most important determinant is skeletal muscle.

If a make-believe human skeleton greeted you on the street, would you recognize it as a normal human?—No.

Consider that skeleton, but also include the human internal organs placed inside the chest wall and body cavities. Does it yet have normal human appearance?—No. Add skin over the bones and organs: still not human.

Return to the image of a skeleton and add the organs, a moderate amount of fat, and skin. Note that the organs and fat droop out of the skin to make the surface appear like melting glue.

Return to the image of the skeleton once more. Now add only well-developed muscles—no organs, no skin, no fat. Note that the resulting shape appears almost identical to the silhouette and contour of a human being. Add the finishing touches of some fat, skin, and organs and you have the appearance of a normal human being.

There is an important lesson to be learned from this demonstration: For improving the body's shape, only muscle and fat can be practically modified. Both are important. Most figure problems are a matter of excess fat *and* inadequate muscle. To lose fat *and* muscle is a serious insult to a woman's appearance and health. Muscle is required to maintain firmness, support overlying fat and skin, flatten puckers, and control posture.

—Ken Hutchins

When you gain muscle, even though your fat weight remains the same, you get leaner in the sense that your body fat becomes a smaller percentage of your overall weight. Conversely, when you lose fat your muscle mass becomes a relatively higher percentage of your body weight. When you both lose fat and gain muscle on the same program, the overall change in body composition and physical appearance can be enormous.

Thus, the ultimate aim of a proper diet and exercise program should be to allow you to lose fat while increasing muscle mass—which is exactly what the Fat-to-Muscle Makeover program does so well!

MUSCLES BURN EXTRA CALORIES

It always amazes me how much food a muscular bodybuilder can eat without gaining fat. Of course, the reason for this is that most champion bodybuilders have extremely low levels of fat and high levels of muscle. Only 8–10 percent of a champion female body-builder's body weight might be fat, compared to 26 percent for the average woman. Much of the champion's weight comes from her muscle.

Unlike fat, muscle contains a large number of capillaries—the tiny vessels that transport blood rich in oxygen throughout the body. This oxygen is used by the muscles to produce the energy necessary for muscular contraction. Fat does not have to work, so it does not need an extensive capillary system. More simply, the muscles are the engines of the body, and fat goes along for the ride. Muscle constantly requires calories for energy; fat never contracts and is actually the product of stored calories. Therefore, it makes sense that a person with a lot of muscle will be able to consume more calories without gaining fat, because her body composition has predisposed her to needing more calories, even at rest.

SHERYL SIMPSON, AGE 31

"ALL MY FRIENDS NOTICED THE CHANGE. I FEEL SO GOOD. THE PROGRAM GOT ME INTO PEAK CONDITION. IT'S WORTH THE PAIN TO FEEL THIS GREAT."

Lost 10¾ pounds of fat and trimmed 2¼ inches off her waist, 1⅜ inches off her hips, 2 inches off her thighs in *six* weeks!

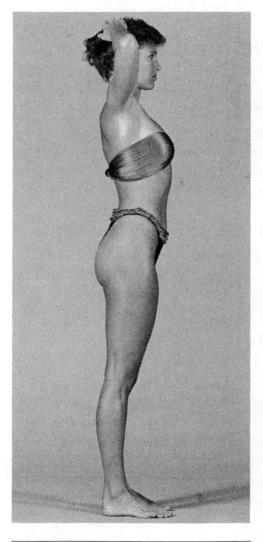

BEFORE
Six-Week Fat-to-Muscle Makeover.

AFTER
Six-Week Fat-to-Muscle Makeover.

When you increase your muscle size, you also increase your body's caloric needs. If these caloric needs aren't met, the body turns to fat stores for energy. The Makeover program works because it builds muscle while reducing your caloric intake, so your body loses fat and gains shapely, strong muscle.

DETERMINING YOUR BODY FAT PERCENTAGE

You should now be convinced that improving your muscle-fat ratio is a key element in enhancing your physical beauty. But how do you determine the amount of fat you have on your body?

There are no direct ways to measure the amount of fat on your body. But there are a number of indirect methods such as underwater weighing, potassium-40 studies, X-ray findings, ultrasound waves, and electrical impedance analysis. All of these methods require special equipment and expertise and can be time-consuming and expensive.

A simpler way to determine percentage of body fat is to use skin-fold measurements. Skin-fold measurements involve gently pinching and pulling the subcutaneous (beneath-the-skin) fat away from the body in various locations and measuring the thickness of the fat with spring-loaded calipers. These measurements are then used in a prediction equation that takes into account sex, age, and state of training to determine your percentage of body fat.

Illustrated details of how to use skin-fold calipers, along with all the charts and graphs to determine your body fat percentage, are found in Chapter 6 of my book *The Nautilus Diet.* You can, however, get a fair estimate of your percentage of body fat by using the pinch test.

THE PINCH TEST

Have a friend do the pinching and measuring. You cannot measure your own skin fold.

1 ▪ Let your right arm hang down at your side.

2 ▪ Have your friend locate the skin-fold site on the back of your upper arm midway between the shoulder and the elbow.

3 ▪ Have your friend grasp a vertical fold of skin between thumb and first finger and pull the skin and fat away from the arm, making sure the fold does not include any muscle, just skin and fat. Practice may be needed in pinching and pulling the skin until there is no muscle included.

4 ▪ Measure with a ruler the thickness of the skin fold to the nearest quarter of an inch, being sure to measure only the distance between the thumb and the finger.

Sometimes the outer portion of the skin fold is thicker than the flesh grasped between the fingers. To avoid this, make sure the fold is level with the side of the thumb. Do not press the ruler against the skin fold. This will flatten it out and make it appear thicker than it really is.

5 ▪ Take two separate measurements of skin-fold thickness, releasing the skin between measurements, and recording the average of the two.

6 ▪ Estimate percentage of body fat from the chart.

ESTIMATED PERCENTAGE OF BODY FAT

TRICEPS SKIN-FOLD THICKNESS	PERCENT FAT WOMEN	MEN
¼ inch	8–13	5–9
½ inch	13–18	9–13
¾ inch	18–23	13–18
1 inch	23–28	18–22
1½ inches	28–33	22–27
2 inches	33–38	27–32
2½ inches	38–43	32–37

MAKEOVER MEASUREMENTS

Each of the ninety women who went through the Fat-to-Muscle Makeover was measured before beginning the program and after its completion. I suggest you take your own before-and-after measurements to see how successful your makeover has been and enter them on a chart (see pages 41–42).

1 ▪ Measure your weight and height. If possible, use a balance-type height-weight scale such as the type found in medical offices.
2 ▪ Take circumference measurements at seven points: both upper arms, the chest, waist, hips, and both thighs.
3 ▪ Measure body-fat percentage, using either skin-fold calipers (your health club or training facility probably has a pair), or the pinch test. If you have access to calipers, have someone experienced at using them measure three points: the back of the arm, above the hipbone, and on the front of the thigh. Apply the sum of these three measurements to a nomograph to calculate your

body fat percentage. Refer to Chapter 6 of *The Nautilus Diet* to find complete instructions and the appropriate nomograph.

4 ■ Determine total fat loss by multiplying percentage of body fat times body weight for the before-and-after tests. (Note: using skin-fold calipers provides more precise numbers than the pinch test.) For instance, if you weighed 130 pounds with 30 percent body fat at the start of the program, that's 39 pounds of fat. If you completed the program at 120 pounds and 20 percent body fat, that's 24 pounds of fat. The difference between 39 and 24 is 15 pounds of total fat lost.

5 ■ Calculate the amount of muscle gained by subtracting the total weight lost from the total fat lost. In the example cited above, fat lost equaled 15 pounds, weight lost equaled 10 pounds—meaning 5 pounds of muscle were gained.

MAKEOVER MEASUREMENTS

NAME _____ AGE _____

DATE: _____ _____

SKIN-FOLD MEASUREMENTS

	Before	After	Difference
Triceps			
Hip			
Thigh			
Total			
Percentage			
Fat pounds			

SCALE WEIGHT

Before	After	Difference

CIRCUMFERENCE MEASUREMENTS

	Before	After	Inches Lost
Right arm			
Left arm			
Chest			
Waist			
Hips			
Right thigh			
Left thigh			

FAT LOST _____

MUSCLE GAINED _____

MAKEOVER PHOTOGRAPHS

Take full-body photographs—like the ones you see in this book—of yourself in a bikini or one-piece bathing suit, before and after the Makeover program.

When starting out on your Makeover program, you'll be tempted to skip this step—but don't. You'll regret it later if you do. When you've accomplished your fat-loss goal, you'll want to see this evidence of your accomplishment.

Follow these instructions:

1 ■ Position yourself several feet in front of an uncluttered background.
2 ■ Stand far enough away from the camera so that your entire body is in the picture.
3 ■ Use the same bathing suit, facial expression, hairstyle, and body position for both the before and the after photo sessions.

ANN DEMAREST, AGE 27

"I USED TO HAVE TO INHALE TO ZIP CERTAIN PANTS AND SKIRTS. NOT ANYMORE! EVERYTHING IS LOOSE. THIS PROGRAM CAME ALONG AT THE PERFECT TIME."

Lost 20¼ pounds of fat and trimmed 5¼ inches off her waist, 2⅛ inches off her hips, 5⅜ inches off her thighs in *six* weeks!

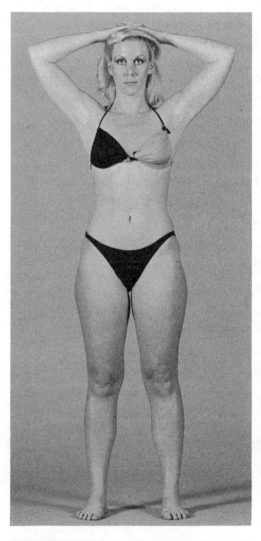
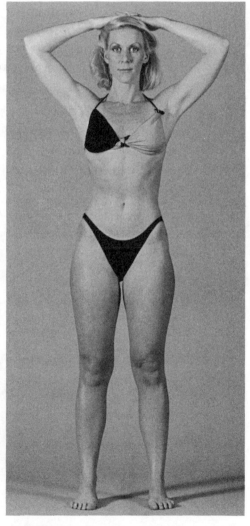

BEFORE
Six-Week Fat-to-Muscle Makeover.

AFTER
Six-Week Fat-to-Muscle Makeover.

4 ▪ Pose in three directions: front, back, and side, with your hands on top of your head in each shot, and feet spaced evenly.

5 ▪ Use black-and-white film, preferably.

You will be amazed at the difference in your appearance after just six weeks. You'll even be excited enough to show your before-and-after photographs to your friends.

THE NEXT STEP

Although tests and measurements—as well as muscle and fat physiology—can be confusing, the bottom line is this: if you have more than ½ inch of fat (skin-fold thickness) on the back of your upper arm, then you are a prime candidate for the Six-Week Fat-to-Muscle Makeover.

You need more muscle and less fat. You need proper exercise and proper diet.

Getting your diet in order is the next step, as you'll see in Part II.

PART II
▪DIETING▪

4

▪ FAT-TO-MUSCLE MAKEOVER DIET ▪

The Fat-to-Muscle Makeover Diet is divided into three two-week segments. Weeks 1 and 2 provide 1,200 calories each day. Weeks 3 and 4 provide 1,100 calories each day; and weeks 5 and 6 provide 1,000 calories. In other words, the calories get fewer with each two-week period.

This descending-calorie plan insures against the symptoms that often occur when calorie intake is drastically reduced: an uncontrollable appetite followed by binging, a quickly tiring body, and the triggering of the system's survival mechanism that preserves fat instead of burning it.

The calories for each day of the Fat-to-Muscle Makeover Diet are selected from the four basic food groups: meat (poultry and fish);

milk (and other dairy products); fruits and vegetables; and breads and cereals. The daily menus adhere to an approximate breakdown of 50 percent carbohydrates, 30 percent fats, and 20 percent proteins. (See below, Daily Guidelines for the Makeover Diet.)

DAILY GUIDELINES FOR THE MAKEOVER DIET.

FOOD GROUP	WEEKS 1 AND 2 1,200 CALORIES	WEEKS 3 AND 4 1,100 CALORIES	WEEKS 5 AND 6 1,000 CALORIES
Meat	3 servings, or a total of 7 oz. cooked weight	2+ servings, or a total of 6 oz. cooked weight	2 servings or a total of 5 oz. cooked weight
Milk	2 cups fortified skim milk	2 cups fortified skim milk	2 cups fortified skim milk
Fruits & vegetables	4 servings	4 servings	3½ servings
Breads & cereals	4 servings	4 servings	4 servings
Other	1 serving	½ serving	0 serving

Notes on serving sizes:

Meat: Choose lean, well-trimmed meats: beef, veal, lamb or pork. Remove the skin from poultry. You may substitute one egg for one serving of meat. One ounce of lean meat equals 60 calories.

Milk: Two cups of milk means two 8-ounce measuring cups. One cup of skim milk equals 100 calories. If you're allergic to milk, substitute plain low-fat or nonfat yogurt for milk.

Fruits and vegetables: One fruit serving equals one medium fruit, two small fruits, ½ banana, ¼ cantaloupe, 10 to 12 grapes or cherries, 1 cup fresh berries or ½ cup fresh, canned or frozen unsweetened fruit or fruit juice. Include one citrus fruit or other good source of vitamin C daily. One fruit or vegetable serving equals 50 to 75 calories. One vegetable serving equals ½ cup cooked or 1 cup raw. Include a leafy vegetable or other good source of vitamin A at least every other day.

Breads and cereals: One serving equals one slice of bread; one small dinner roll; ½ cup cooked cereal; noodles, macaroni, spaghetti, rice or cornmeal; 1 ounce (approximately 1 cup) ready-to-eat un-sweetened, iron-fortified cereal. One bread or cereal serving equals 75 calories.

Other: One serving equals 1 teaspoon butter, margarine or oil; 6 nuts; 2 teaspoons salad dressing.

The American Heart Association recommends that daily intake of fats not exceed 30 percent. The fat content of the diet is kept at 30 percent for this and one other reason. Research shows that eating a diet with too little fat does not provide satiety, making it more difficult to avoid cheating.

SIMPLE AND SPECIFIC

Another big plus of the Makeover Diet is its simplicity. Research establishes that most dieters prefer specific recommendations, as opposed to general guidelines. Research also reveals that most dieters like the idea of consuming the same foods each day for breakfast, and having only a few choices for lunch. Dinner, however, should offer ample variety.

Every day for six weeks you are given a choice of two approx-imately 250-calorie breakfasts.

Lunch is limited to two approximately 350-calorie menus which stay the same for the entire six weeks. However, during weeks 5 and 6 a Sunday brunch, which may replace breakfast and lunch, is introduced.

Dinner offers the most variety. After a two-week introduction to seven approximately 400-calorie meals, an alternate meal suggestion will be added for weeks 3 and 4 and again for weeks 5 and 6. You'll never get bored with these low-calorie but highly nutritious meals, because they've all been tried and tested in 1986 and 1987 with women just like you.

Furthermore, the Makeover Diet won't leave you starving between meals. You'll always be provided with midafternoon and late-night snacks.

Lastly, the diet comes equipped with shopping lists of all foods you'll need to have handy each week. These will make your trips to the supermarket more efficient.

CHECK WITH YOUR DOCTOR

Before you begin the six-week program, make sure your doctor knows you are about to modify both your eating and exercising habits. Show him a copy of this book so he knows exactly what is involved. He'll probably want to give you a thorough physical examination if he hasn't done so in the last year.

There are a few women who should *not* try the Fat-to-Muscle Makeover program. For example, teenagers and children; pregnant women; nursing mothers; women with certain types of heart, liver, and kidney disease; diabetics; and women suffering from some types of arthritis. Other women should follow the Six-Week Fat-to-Muscle Makeover only with their physician's specific guidance and recommendations. Play it safe by consulting your doctor.

MOVING INTO ACTION

The next five chapters cover all the details and how-to's of the Fat-to-Muscle Makeover Diet. Let's get started.

5

▪ WEEKS 1 AND 2 ▪

Hawaiian Chicken, Zesty Spaghetti, Beef Oriental, and the other dishes you are about to enjoy will make you forget that you are on a diet. This sensible eating plan is really a calorie-management program. You may have to resist certain temptations, foods in which you've customarily indulged, but you'll be surprised at how satisfied you feel.

"This is the only diet I've been on in my life where I have not been hungry," remarked Ginger Masingill, a 37-year-old mother of three. "I used to get headaches on other diets."

Ginger's results are among the best on record. She dropped 26 pounds during her Makeover in DeLand. "A lot of it has been willpower," she commented, "but it hasn't been torture."

The menus in this Makeover Diet are designed for maximum effectiveness and nutritional value. They feature tasty dishes and easy-to-follow recipes. For best results, follow them exactly as directed.

Remember that this is not an allotment of calories, but a blueprint. Consume every calorie spelled out in the diet. *If you attempt to accelerate your progress by eating fewer calories, you'll be slowing your rate of fat loss, not boosting it.*

A practitioner of our ten-week Nautilus Diet experimentally put a group of his clients on fewer calories than directed. The fat-loss results of this group did not match those of their counterparts — who were eating 400 more calories per day.

You want to make your body an efficient fat burner. Inadequate caloric intake will trigger starvation signals, lowering metabolism and causing preservation of fat. Best results are achieved by following the blueprint — *exactly!*

It is also best not to skip meals or carry over calories from one meal to the next. However, subtracting foods from lunch and dinner to use as snacks between meals is allowed, especially during weeks 5 and 6.

Substitute only as absolutely necessary. Those allergic to milk may substitute 1 ounce of cheese or 1 cup of low-fat yogurt for 1 cup of milk. Vegetarians may substitute one egg or a cup of cooked dried beans or peas for one meat serving.

Most of the recipes in Chapter 8 make one serving. If other family members are going to be enjoying the same foods, multiply by the number of people you are feeding, or more if they desire larger portions.

GINGER MASINGILL, AGE 37

"MY PARENTS NOT ONLY NOTICED THAT I LOOKED BETTER, BUT THEY COULD EVEN TELL THAT I HAD MORE ENERGY — AND KEEPING UP WITH THREE KIDS REQUIRES LOTS OF ENERGY. I APPRECIATE FEELING BETTER AS WELL AS LOOKING BETTER."

Lost 26 pounds of fat and trimmed 3⅝ inches off her waist, 3½ inches off her hips, 4½ inches off her thighs in *six* weeks!

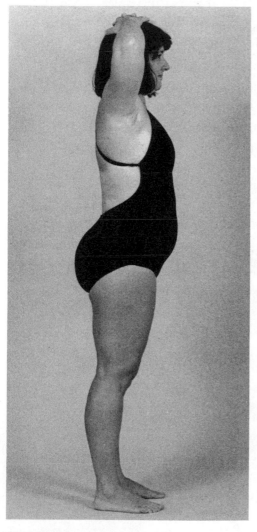
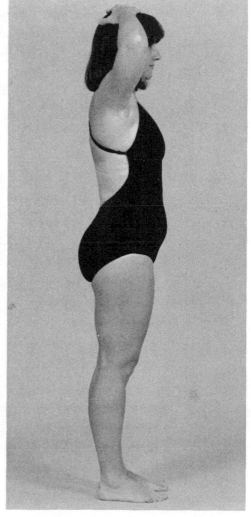

BEFORE
Six-Week Fat-to-Muscle Makeover.

AFTER
Six-Week Fat-to-Muscle Makeover.

COOKING PARTY

You may also want to try a time-saving idea that some of the Florida women used. They'd cook a supply of meals on the weekends, which they would then freeze and reheat at the appropriate time.

And they had fun doing it. Instead of inviting over a friend and serving calorie-intensive snacks, two or more women would get together for a Sunday afternoon cooking party. This saved time when needed most, during hectic weekdays of trying to keep up with household, motherhood, and job responsibilities.

The Zesty Spaghetti, Beef Oriental, and chicken dishes freeze well. Cooked fish, however, is not very tasty once it has been frozen. But neither does it take long to cook.

It will also be helpful to cook and freeze larger quantities of marinara sauce and brown rice.

Even if you enjoy cooking each night, have one or two emergency dinners stashed in the freezer. There will always be occasions when you just don't have the time. Even if it is not the night of the week for the dinner available in the freezer, go ahead and eat it. This is far better than stopping for a hamburger and fries, or skipping dinner all together.

THREE IMPORTANT GUIDELINES

1 ▪ Although the Makeover Diet is well balanced, take *one* multiple-vitamin-with-minerals tablet each day. Make sure that no nutrient listed on the label exceeds 100 percent of the U.S. Recommended Daily Allowance. You are wasting your money if you take high-potency supplements.

2 ■ Give up alcohol entirely until you reach your fat-loss goal. If you feel you must have alcohol in the diet plan, limit it strictly to one drink a day or no more than 150 calories. Add this amount on top of your daily menus and calorie counts and resign yourself to a slower rate of fat loss.

3 ■ Drink at least six to eight glasses of water each day. Water is particularly helpful to dieters because it diminishes feelings of hunger and supplies a sense of satiety. Water also assists your kidneys and gastrointestinal tract in eliminating wastes from your body.

Invariably, the Florida women who achieved the best results — such as Ginger Masingill — were those who consumed the most water. It works.

Ginger found that drinking water through a straw enabled her to drink more. Who knows why, but maybe such a strategy will work for you, too.

START ON A MONDAY

You are about to initiate your Makeover. Once preparation has been completed, begin week 1 on Monday and continue through Sunday. Week 2 is an exact repeat of the first week.

Calories for each food are noted in parentheses. An asterisk (*) preceding a listing indicates that a recipe for that dish may be found in Chapter 8. A shopping list is provided in Chapter 9.

Congratulations on taking this important step. Part III of this book explains the corresponding exercise routine you should employ. Good luck in all phases of your Fat-to-Muscle Makeover.

▪ MENUS ▪

WEEKS 1 AND 2

MONDAY: Total calories, including snacks: 1,198

BREAKFAST: 267 CALORIES

BASIC BREAKFAST #1
Cereal choices (1 ounce
   serving, 110 calories):
Nabisco Shredded Wheat
Kellogg's Frosted Mini-
   Wheats
Kellogg's Nutri-Grain Wheat
   or Corn
Post Grape-Nuts

Ralston Purina Almond
   Delight
Ralston Purina Sun Flakes
   Crispy Wheat & Rice
¾ cup cooked oatmeal,
   sprinkled with cinnamon
   and low-calorie sweetener

Plus

½ cup skim milk (45)
½ cup orange juice (55)
1 slice reduced-calorie bread,
   toasted (40)

1 teaspoon low-calorie
   margarine (17)
Noncaloric beverage

or

BASIC BREAKFAST #2
*Breakfast Shake, recipe #1 (267)

LUNCH: 349 CALORIES

BASIC LUNCH #1
Sandwich (roast beef or tuna):

2 slices reduced-calorie bread (80)

½ tablespoon low-calorie mayonnaise (20)

2 slices tomato (14)

1 lettuce leaf (2)

2 ounces sliced lean roast beef (from the deli) *or*

½ can (6½ ounce size) water-packed tuna (110)

Plus

1 cup skim milk (90)

⅔ cup one of the following:
blueberries (33) or
sliced strawberries (33) or
applesauce (33) or
diced cantaloupe (33)

Noncaloric beverage

or

BASIC LUNCH #2
*Chef salad, recipe #2 (169)

1 slice reduced-calorie bread (40)

1 teaspoon low-calorie margarine (17)

Plus

1 cup skim milk (90)

⅔ cup one of the following:
blueberries (33) or
sliced strawberries (33) or
applesauce (33) or
diced cantaloupe (33)

Noncaloric beverage

SNACK: 60 CALORIES

1 whole graham cracker (4 sections) (60)

1 cup hot tea or coffee (0)

or

1 cup low-sodium bouillon (12)

4 saltines (48)

DINNER: 404 CALORIES

*Hawaiian Chicken, recipe #3 (215)
*Grilled Tomato, recipe #4 (59)

1 ear corn (5 inches), fresh or frozen (70)

Salad:
  1 cup fresh young spinach leaves (9)
  5 fresh mushrooms, sliced (5)

1 tablespoon diet Italian dressing (6)

1 slice reduced-calorie bread (40)

Noncaloric beverage

SNACK: 118 CALORIES

½ cup ice milk (100)

½ slice canned pineapple, juice-packed (18)

TUESDAY: Total calories, including snacks: 1,200

BREAKFAST: 267 CALORIES

Basic Breakfast #1

or

Basic Breakfast #2

LUNCH: 349 CALORIES

Basic Lunch #1

or

Basic Lunch #2

SNACK: 60 CALORIES

1 whole graham cracker (4 sections) (60)	1 cup hot tea or coffee (0)

or

1 cup low-sodium bouillon (12)	4 saltines (48)

DINNER: 404 CALORIES

*Chicken Chowder, recipe #5 (205)

½ acorn squash (4 inch diameter) (86),
  baked with 2 teaspoons low-calorie margarine (34);
  to squash add 1½ tablespoons raisins (39),
  sprinkle with cinnamon and ginger

1 slice reduced-calorie bread (40)

Noncaloric beverage

SNACK: 120 CALORIES

1 whole graham cracker (4 sections) (60)

⅔ cup skim milk (60)

WEDNESDAY: Total calories, including snacks: 1,203

BREAKFAST: 267 CALORIES

Basic Breakfast #1

or

Basic Breakfast #2

LUNCH: 349 CALORIES

Basic Lunch #1

or

Basic Lunch #2

SNACK: 60 CALORIES

1 whole graham cracker (4 sections) (60)

1 cup hot tea or coffee (0)

or

1 cup low-sodium bouillon (12)

4 saltines (48)

DINNER: 417 CALORIES

*Zesty Spaghetti, recipe #6
(298)

Salad:

1 cup fresh young spinach
leaves (9)
5 fresh mushrooms, sliced
(5)

1 tablespoon diet Italian
dressing (6)

1 slice reduced-calorie bread
(40)
2 teaspoons low-calorie
margarine (34)

½ cup sliced strawberries (25)
Noncaloric beverage

SNACK: 110 CALORIES

1 medium peach (6 ounces,
2¾ inch diameter) *or* ½
cup canned pears, juice-
packed (50)

1 whole graham cracker (4
sections) (60)

THURSDAY: Total calories, including snacks: 1,207

BREAKFAST: 267 CALORIES

Basic Breakfast #1

or

Basic Breakfast #2

LUNCH: 349 CALORIES

Basic Lunch #1

or

Basic Lunch #2

SNACK: 60 CALORIES

1 whole graham cracker (4 sections) (60)

1 cup hot tea or coffee (0)

or

1 cup low-sodium bouillon (12)

4 saltines (48)

DINNER: 401 CALORIES

*Stuffed Potato, recipe #7
(208)

1 cup French-style green
beans, steamed (31)

1 ear corn (5 inches), fresh or
frozen (70)

1 teaspoon low-calorie
margarine (17)

1 slice reduced-calorie bread
(40)

1 slice canned pineapple,
juice-packed (35)

Noncaloric beverage

SNACK: 130 CALORIES

1 ounce part-skim mozzarella
cheese (90)

1 slice reduced-calorie bread
(40)

Noncaloric beverage

FRIDAY: Total calories, including snacks: 1,201

BREAKFAST: 267 CALORIES

Basic Breakfast #1

or

Basic Breakfast #2

LUNCH: 349 CALORIES

Basic Lunch #1

or

Basic Lunch #2

SNACK: 60 CALORIES

1 whole graham cracker (4 sections) (60)	1 cup hot tea or coffee (0)

or

1 cup low-sodium bouillon (12)	4 saltines (48)

DINNER: 400 CALORIES

6 ounces vegetable juice cocktail (35)

*Ginger Fish, recipe #8 (161)

1 small potato (2½ inch diameter, 4½ ounces), baked (90)

1 cup chopped broccoli, steamed (40)

1 slice reduced-calorie bread (40)

2 teaspoons low-calorie margarine (34)

Noncaloric beverage

SNACK: 125 CALORIES

½ cup ice milk (100)

½ cup sliced strawberries (25)

SATURDAY: Total calories, including snacks: 1,205

BREAKFAST: 267 CALORIES

Basic Breakfast #1

or

Basic Breakfast #2

LUNCH: 349 CALORIES

Basic Lunch #1

or

Basic Lunch #2

SNACK: 60 CALORIES

1 whole graham cracker (4 sections) (60)

1 cup hot tea or coffee (0)

or

1 cup low-sodium bouillon (12)

4 saltines (48)

DINNER: 407 CALORIES

*Orange Chicken, recipe #9 (198)

½ cup steamed brown rice (116)

1 cup French-style green beans, steamed (31)

Salad:

⅓ sliced banana (medium) (34)

½ tablespoon raisins (13)

1 teaspoon low-calorie mayonnaise (13)

served on 1 lettuce leaf (2)

Noncaloric beverage

SNACK: 122 CALORIES

Remaining banana, sliced (67)

½ cup sliced strawberries (25)

½ graham cracker (2 sections) (30)

Noncaloric beverage

SUNDAY: Total calories, including snacks: 1,201

BREAKFAST: 267 CALORIES

Basic Breakfast #1

or

Basic Breakfast #2

LUNCH: 349 CALORIES

Basic Lunch #1

or

Basic Lunch #2

SNACK: 60 CALORIES

1 whole graham cracker (4 sections) (60)	1 cup hot tea or coffee (0)

or

1 cup low-sodium bouillon (12)	4 saltines (48)

DINNER: 407 CALORIES

6 ounces vegetable juice
   cocktail (35)
*Beef Oriental, recipe #10
   (241)

½ cup steamed brown rice
   (116)

Salad:
   1 cup chopped lettuce (9)

1 tablespoon diet Italian
   dressing (6)

Noncaloric beverage

SNACK: 118 CALORIES

1 medium peach (6 ounces,
   2¾ inch diameter) *or* ½
   cup canned pears, juice-
   packed (50)

¾ cup skim milk (68)

6

▪WEEKS 3 AND 4▪

Slight modifications have been incorporated into the diet during weeks 3 and 4.

First, the daily calories drop from 1,200 to 1,100. Most of the missing calories come from your snacks and evening meals.

Second, one optional evening meal—Scallop Dinner—is provided as an alternative to any of the seven you would like to replace. If you don't like Ginger Fish, for example, you may want to substitute the Scallop Dinner—recipe #11 in Chapter 8. Or you may simply enjoy knowing that you now have some flexibility in your evening meal selection.

If you don't need additional variety, and most women will not, then keep your evening meals for weeks 3 and 4 in the same order as the first two weeks.

You might wonder why we employ a strategy of minimized changes. The reason is that you need to master the recipes. Every component of every meal must be measured or weighed. Make sure that you have an accurate scale and measuring cups. This will seem laborious at first, but it soon becomes second nature.

You must hit the calorie targets within a very few calories: 1,200 the first two weeks, 1,100 during weeks 3 and 4, and 1,000 the final two weeks. Changing the menu creates a margin for error, which could derail our descending-calorie plan.

Your success depends on the degree to which you are able to stick to the diet. And that is made as simple as it possibly can be.

LEARN TO HANDLE LAPSES

How closely were you able to follow the diet during the first two weeks? Dieting success depends on identifying self-defeating attitudes and devising effective strategies to prevent a relapse, according to Dr. Kelly D. Brownell, a psychologist at the University of Pennsylvania. Dr. Brownell directs a comprehensive weight-control program.

"Some dieters feel that an urge builds and builds and will create havoc unless it is gratified by eating," Dr. Brownell says. "Actually, gratifying an urge by eating makes urges stronger and more frequent. In contrast, letting the urge pass, like the wave rolling in, will weaken it. If you can outlast enough of the urges, they will fade to obscurity. If you can distract yourself for even a few minutes, the urge to eat can fade."

If you were not able to follow the diet exactly, examine the circumstances that caused you to lapse. Identify what psychologists term the *trigger factors.* This will help you avoid similar pitfalls in the future. *Strengthen your resolve.*

Now let's take a look at the menus for weeks 3 and 4.

▪ MENUS ▪
WEEKS 3 AND 4

MONDAY: Total calories, including snacks: 1,093

BREAKFAST: 267 CALORIES

BASIC BREAKFAST #1
Cereal choices (1 ounce
  serving, 110 calories):
Nabisco Shredded Wheat
Kellogg's Frosted Mini
  Wheats
Kellogg's NutriGrain wheat or
  corn
Post Grape Nuts

Ralston Purina Almond
  Delight
Ralston Purina Sun Flakes
  Crispy Wheat & Rice
¾ cup cooked oatmeal,
  sprinkled with cinnamon
  and low-calorie sweetener

Plus

½ cup skim milk (45)
½ cup orange juice (55)1 slice
  reduced-calorie bread,
  toasted (40)

1 teaspoon low-calorie
  margarine (17)
Noncaloric beverage

or

BASIC BREAKFAST #2
*Breakfast Shake, recipe #1 (267)

LUNCH: 349 CALORIES

BASIC LUNCH #1
Sandwich (roast beef or tuna):

2 slices reduced-calorie
bread (80)

½ tablespoon low-calorie
mayonnaise (20)

2 slices tomato (14)

1 lettuce leaf (2)

2 ounces sliced lean roast beef
(from the deli) *or*

½ can (6½ ounce size) water-
packed tuna (110)

Plus

1 cup skim milk (90)

⅔ cup one of the following:
blueberries (33) or
sliced strawberries (33) or
applesauce (33) or
diced cantaloupe (33)

Noncaloric beverage

or

BASIC LUNCH #2
*Chef salad, recipe #2 (169)

1 slice reduced-calorie bread
(40)

1 teaspoon low-calorie
margarine (17)

Plus

1 cup skim milk (90)

⅔ cup one of the following:
blueberries (33) or
sliced strawberries (33) or
applesauce (33) or
diced cantaloupe (33)

Noncaloric beverage

SNACK: 0 CALORIES

1 cup hot tea or coffee (0)

(fruit serving left over from lunch)

DINNER: 359 CALORIES

*Hawaiian Chicken, recipe #3 (215)
2 slices tomato (14)

1 ear corn (5 inches), fresh or frozen (70)

Salad:
  1 cup fresh young spinach leaves (9)
  5 fresh mushrooms, sliced (5)

1 tablespoon diet Italian dressing (6)

1 slice reduced-calorie bread (40)

Noncaloric beverage

SNACK: 118 CALORIES

½ cup ice milk (100)

½ slice canned pineapple, juice-packed (18)

TUESDAY: Total calories, including snacks: 1,099

BREAKFAST: 267 CALORIES

Basic Breakfast #1

or

Basic Breakfast #2

LUNCH: 349 CALORIES

Basic Lunch #1

or

Basic Lunch #2

SNACK: 0 CALORIES

1 cup hot tea or coffee (0)   (fruit serving left over from
                                              lunch)

DINNER: 378 CALORIES

*Chicken Chowder, recipe #5 (205)

½ acorn squash (4 inch diameter) (86), baked with 2 teaspoons low-calorie margarine (34), to squash add ½ tablespoon raisins (13), sprinkle with cinnamon and ginger

1 slice reduced-calorie bread (40)

Noncaloric beverage

SNACK: 105 CALORIES

¾ graham cracker (3 sections) (45)

⅔ cup skim milk (60)

WEDNESDAY: Total calories, including snacks: 1,094

BREAKFAST: 267 CALORIES

Basic Breakfast #1

or

Basic Breakfast #2

LUNCH: 349 CALORIES

Basic Lunch #1

or

Basic Lunch #2

SNACK: 0 CALORIES

1 cup hot tea or
   coffee (0)

(fruit serving left over from
   lunch)

DINNER: 383 CALORIES

*Zesty Spaghetti, recipe #6
(298)

Salad:

1 cup fresh young spinach
leaves (9)
5 fresh mushrooms, sliced
(5)

1 tablespoon diet Italian
dressing (6)

1 slice reduced-calorie bread
(40)

½ cup sliced strawberries (25)
Noncaloric beverage

SNACK: 95 CALORIES

1 medium peach (6 ounces,
2¾ inch diameter) *or* ½
cup canned pears, juice-
packed (50)

¾ graham cracker (3 sections)
(45)

THURSDAY: Total calories, including snacks: 1,100

BREAKFAST: 267 CALORIES

Basic Breakfast #1

or

Basic Breakfast #2

LUNCH: 349 CALORIES

Basic Lunch #1

or

Basic Lunch #2

SNACK: 0 CALORIES

1 cup hot tea or coffee (0)

(fruit serving left over from lunch)

DINNER: 384 CALORIES

*Stuffed Potato, recipe #7 (208)

1 cup French-style green beans, steamed (31)

1 ear corn (5 inches), fresh or frozen (70)

1 slice reduced-calorie bread (40)

1 slice canned pineapple, juice-packed (35)

Noncaloric beverage

SNACK: 100 CALORIES

⅔ ounce part-skim mozzarella cheese (60)

1 slice reduced-calorie bread (40)

Noncaloric beverage

FRIDAY: Total calories, including snacks: 1,107

BREAKFAST: 267 CALORIES

Basic Breakfast #1

or

Basic Breakfast #2

LUNCH: 349 CALORIES

Basic Lunch #1

or

Basic Lunch #2

SNACK: 0 CALORIES

1 cup hot tea or
    coffee (0)

(fruit serving left over from
    lunch)

DINNER: 366 CALORIES

6 ounces vegetable juice
cocktail (35)

*Ginger Fish, recipe #8
(161)

1 small potato (2½ inch
diameter, 4½ ounces),
baked (90)

1 cup chopped broccoli,
steamed (40)

1 slice reduced-calorie bread
(40)

Noncaloric beverage

SNACK: 125 CALORIES

½ cup ice milk (100)

½ cup sliced strawberries (25)

SATURDAY: Total calories, including snacks: 1,102

BREAKFAST: 267 CALORIES

Basic Breakfast #1

or

Basic Breakfast #2

LUNCH: 349 CALORIES

Basic Lunch #1

or

Basic Lunch #2

SNACK: 0 CALORIES

1 cup hot tea or
 coffee (0)

(fruit serving left over from
 lunch)

DINNER: 379 CALORIES

*Orange Chicken, recipe #9
(198)
½ cup steamed brown rice
(116)

½ cup French-style green
beans, steamed (16)

Salad:
⅓ sliced banana (medium)
(34)
1 teaspoon low-calorie
mayonnaise (13)

served on 1 lettuce leaf (2)

Noncaloric beverage

SNACK: 107 CALORIES

Remaining banana, sliced (67)
½ cup sliced strawberries
(25)

¼ graham cracker (1 section)
(15)
Noncaloric beverage

SUNDAY: Total calories, including snacks: 1,099

BREAKFAST: 267 CALORIES

Basic Breakfast #1

or

Basic Breakfast #2

LUNCH: 349 CALORIES

Basic Lunch #1

or

Basic Lunch #2

SNACK: 0 CALORIES

1 cup hot tea or
  coffee (0)

(fruit serving left over from
  lunch)

DINNER: 365 CALORIES

6 ounces vegetable juice
cocktail (35)
*Beef Oriental, recipe #10
Note: Start with only 5
ounces lean round steak.
(183)

½ cup steamed brown rice
(116)

Salad:

1 cup chopped lettuce (9)
1 small stalk celery (4 inches
long), chopped (3)
2 tablespoons grated carrot
(6)

1 slice tomato, chopped (7)
1 tablespoon diet Italian
dressing (6)

Noncaloric beverage

SNACK: 118 CALORIES

1 medium peach (6 ounces,
2¾ inch diameter) *or* ½
cup canned pears, juice-
packed (50)

¾ cup skim milk (68)

7

▪ WEEKS 5 AND 6 ▪

After four weeks of sweat and discipline, you might be curious about how you're doing in comparison to other women who have followed the Makeover Diet. Six pounds was the average weight loss of the Florida women after four weeks, with a normal range of 4 to 8 pounds. In other words, your results would be considered average if you have lost between 4 and 8 pounds.

Perhaps you are disappointed that your weight hasn't plummeted. If you've followed diets in the past that did not include high-quality exercise, you might be accustomed to rapid *weight* loss.

Remember the distinction between *weight* loss and *fat* loss, and the measurement that most interests us—muscle-to-fat ratio (refresh your memory by reviewing Chapter 3).

If you've been following the exercise guidelines that are described in Part III of this book, you should be building muscle. Thus, your fat loss will be significantly greater than your weight loss, and that's a major objective of the Fat-to-Muscle Makeover program.

Just like the Florida women, you should be noticing a big change in the fit of your clothing. Perhaps the best measurement is the tight-pants test. Try on the same pair of tight-fitting pants every week — and see how dramatically they loosen.

CHECK FOR ERRORS

But if your weight loss at the beginning of week 5 is less than 4 pounds, ask yourself the following questions:

- Are you following the menus exactly as directed? Are you sure you're not consuming too many calories? Remember, all calories count.
- Are your weighing practices consistent? One or two pounds of additional clothing or different shoes can make a big difference. And weighing at different times of the day can influence the scale.
- Did your last weighing occur just before the start of your menstrual period? Many women have a tendency to retain water during the week preceding their period. If this is the case, this water fluctuation will balance itself out over the long run.

DESCENDING THE CALORIES

You are at full throttle during the final two weeks, exercise at the maximum and food intake at the minimum — 1,000 calories. This is as low as the daily calories go during the six-week program. Also, you can add another new dinner — Pork Chop — to your selection of evening meals. It's listed in Chapter 8.

As an additional bonus, a Sunday Brunch has been devised: a scrambled egg and three pancakes.

Here are the final two weeks of menus. Follow them to the letter — and your Makeover will be an astonishing success!

▪ MENUS ▪
WEEKS 5 AND 6

MONDAY: Total calories, including snacks: 1,004

BREAKFAST: 267 CALORIES

BASIC BREAKFAST #1

Cereal choices (1 ounce serving, 110 calories):
Nabisco Shredded Wheat
Kellogg's Frosted Mini Wheats
Kellogg's NutriGrain wheat or corn
Post Grape Nuts

Ralston Purina Almond Delight
Ralston Purina Sun Flakes Crispy Wheat & Rice
¾ cup cooked oatmeal, sprinkled with cinnamon and low-calorie sweetener

Plus

½ cup skim milk (45)
½ cup orange juice (55)
1 slice reduced-calorie bread, toasted (40)

1 teaspoon low-calorie margarine (17)
Noncaloric beverage

or

BASIC BREAKFAST #2
*Breakfast Shake, recipe #1 (267)

LUNCH: 349 CALORIES

BASIC LUNCH #1

Sandwich (roast beef or tuna):
  2 slices reduced-calorie
    bread (80)
  ½ tablespoon low-calorie
    mayonnaise (20)
  2 slices tomato (14)

1 lettuce leaf (2)
2 ounces sliced lean roast beef
  (from the deli) *or*
½ can (6½ ounce size) water-
  packed tuna (110)

Plus

1 cup skim milk (90)
⅔ cup one of the following:
  blueberries (33) or
  sliced strawberries (33) or
  applesauce (33) or
  diced cantaloupe (33)

Noncaloric beverage

or

BASIC LUNCH #2

*Chef salad, recipe #2 (169)
1 slice reduced-calorie bread
  (40)

1 teaspoon low-calorie
  margarine (17)

Plus

1 cup skim milk (90)
⅔ cup one of the following:
  blueberries (33) or
  sliced strawberries (33) or
  applesauce (33) or
  diced cantaloupe (33)

Noncaloric beverage

SNACK: 0 CALORIES

1 cup hot tea or
coffee (0)

(fruit serving left over from
lunch)

DINNER: 320 CALORIES

*Hawaiian Chicken, recipe
#3 Note: use only ½
pineapple slice on chicken.
(198)

2 slices tomato (14)
3 ounces new potatoes,
steamed (48)

Salad:

1 cup fresh young spinach
leaves (9)
5 fresh mushrooms, sliced
(5)
1 slice reduced-calorie bread
(40)

1 tablespoon diet Italian
dressing (6)

Noncaloric beverage

SNACK: 68 CALORIES

¼ cup ice milk (50)
½ slice canned pineapple,
juice-packed (18)

TUESDAY: Total calories, including snacks: 1,003

BREAKFAST: 267 CALORIES

Basic Breakfast #1

or

Basic Breakfast #2

LUNCH: 349 CALORIES

Basic Lunch #1

or

Basic Lunch #2

SNACK: 0 CALORIES

1 cup hot tea or coffee (0)

(fruit serving left over from lunch)

DINNER: 342 CALORIES

*Chicken Chowder, recipe #5
  (205)

½ cup carrots (sliced crosswise ¼–½ inch thick), steamed until crisp-tender (24) with ½ tablespoon raisins (13), sprinkled with cinnamon and ginger

1 slice reduced-calorie bread (40)

⅔ cup skim milk (60)

SNACK: 45 CALORIES

¾ graham cracker (3 sections) (45)

1 cup hot tea or coffee (0)

WEDNESDAY: Total calories, including snacks: 1,004

BREAKFAST: 267 CALORIES

Basic Breakfast #1

or

Basic Breakfast #2

LUNCH: 349 CALORIES

Basic Lunch #1

or

Basic Lunch #2

SNACK: 0 CALORIES

1 cup hot tea or
   coffee (0)

(fruit serving left over from
   lunch)

DINNER: 338 CALORIES

*Zesty Spaghetti, recipe #6,
  prepared with only ½ ounce
  mozarella (253)

Salad:

1 cup fresh young spinach
  leaves (9)
5 fresh mushrooms, sliced
  (5)

1 tablespoon diet Italian
  dressing (6)

1 slice reduced-calorie bread
  (40)

½ cup sliced strawberries (25)
Noncaloric beverage

SNACK: 50 CALORIES

1 medium peach (6 ounces,
  2¾ inch diameter) *or*

½ cup canned pears, juice-
  packed (50)

THURSDAY: Total calories, including snacks: 1,005

BREAKFAST: 267 CALORIES

Basic Breakfast #1

or

Basic Breakfast #2

LUNCH: 349 CALORIES

Basic Lunch #1

or

Basic Lunch #2

SNACK: 0 CALORIES

1 cup hot tea or   (fruit serving left over from
   coffee (0)   lunch)

DINNER: 344 CALORIES

*Stuffed Potato, recipe #7
(208)
1 cup French-style green
beans, steamed (31)
1 ear corn (5 inches), fresh or
frozen (70)

1 slice canned pineapple,
juice-packed (35)
Noncaloric beverage

SNACK: 45 CALORIES

¾ graham cracker (3 sections)
(45)

1 cup hot tea or coffee (0)

FRIDAY: Total calories, including snacks: 1,003

BREAKFAST: 267 CALORIES

Basic Breakfast #1

or

Basic Breakfast #2

LUNCH: 349 CALORIES

Basic Lunch #1

or

Basic Lunch #2

SNACK: 0 CALORIES

1 cup hot tea or coffee (0)

(fruit serving left over from lunch)

DINNER: 324 CALORIES

6 ounces vegetable juice
   cocktail (35)
*Ginger Fish, recipe #8
   (161)
3 ounces new potatoes,
   steamed (48)

1 cup chopped broccoli,
   steamed (40)
1 slice reduced-calorie bread
   (40)
Noncaloric beverage

SNACK: 63 CALORIES

¼ cup ice milk (50)

¼ cup sliced strawberries (13)

SATURDAY: Total calories, including snacks: 999

BREAKFAST: 267 CALORIES

Basic Breakfast #1

or

Basic Breakfast #2

LUNCH: 349 CALORIES

Basic Lunch #1

or

Basic Lunch #2

SNACK: 0 CALORIES

1 cup hot tea or coffee (0)

(fruit serving left over from lunch)

DINNER: 303 CALORIES

*Orange Chicken, recipe #9 (198)

½ cup French-style green beans, steamed (16)

Salad:

⅓ sliced banana (medium) (34)

served on 1 lettuce leaf (2)

1 teaspoon low-calorie mayonnaise (13)

1 slice reduced-calorie bread (40)

Noncaloric beverage

SNACK: 80 CALORIES

Remaining banana, sliced (67)
¼ cup sliced strawberries (13)

Noncaloric beverage

SUNDAY: Total calories, including snacks: 1,003 or 999 (with Brunch)

BREAKFAST: 267 CALORIES

Basic Breakfast #1

or

Basic Breakfast #2

LUNCH: 349 CALORIES

Basic Lunch #1

or

Basic Lunch #2

Or

EGG AND PANCAKE SUNDAY BRUNCH: 579 CALORIES

(replaces breakfast and lunch)
  1 egg scrambled, nonstick pan (82)
  3 pancakes (4 inch diameter), from mix, with egg and milk (180)
  3 tablespoons syrup (120)

2 medium slices bacon (85)
1 slice reduced-calorie bread (40)
1 teaspoon diet margarine (17)
½ cup orange juice (55)

SNACK: 0 CALORIES

1 cup hot tea or coffee (0)
(If you choose the Brunch,
   add one fruit serving from
   the Basic lunch) (33)

DINNER: 337 CALORIES

*Beef Oriental, recipe #10
   Note: Start with only 5
   ounces lean round steak.
   (183)

½ cup steamed brown rice
   (116)

Salad:
   1 cup chopped lettuce (9)
   1 small celery stalk (4 inches
      long), chopped (3)
   2 tablespoons grated carrot
      (6)

2 slices tomato, chopped (14)
1 tablespoon diet Italian
   dressing (6)

Noncaloric beverage

SNACK: 50 CALORIES

1 medium peach (6 ounces,
   2¾ inch diameter) *or* ½
   cup canned pears, juice-
   packed (50)

8

▪RECIPES ▪

Recipes do not have to be complicated, nor require a long preparation time, to be delicious and satisfying. In fact, all the recipes in this chapter are relatively easy to fix, tasty, and filling.

The recipes are numbered consecutively to correspond with their appearance in the text.

RECIPE #1

BREAKFAST SHAKE

INGREDIENTS:

½ large banana (9¾ inches long), frozen
½ cup orange juice
½ cup skim milk

2 tablespoons wheat germ
½ teaspoon vanilla extract
1 teaspoon vegetable oil
2 ice cubes (optional)

Peel banana, cut in half and wrap halves separately in aluminum foil or other airtight wrapper. Freeze overnight. The next day, combine all ingredients, except ice cubes, in blender container or food processor. Cover; blend until smooth. If a thicker consistency is desired, add ice cubes and blend until thick and creamy. Serve immediately.

YIELD: 1 serving
CALORIES: 267

RECIPE #2

CHEF SALAD

INGREDIENTS:

1½ cups shredded lettuce

2 slices tomato, chopped

6 slices large cucumber (2⅛ inch diameter)

1 tablespoon chopped green onion

2 tablespoons sliced celery

2 tablespoons grated carrot

2 rings green pepper (3 inch diameter, sliced ¼ inch thick)

Plus choice of one:

2 ounces chicken, skinned and roasted; *or*

2 ounces turkey, skinned and roasted; *or*

1½ ounces ham (trimmed of excess fat), baked; *or*

1 ounce cheese:
   Swiss or
   Monterey Jack or
   part-skim mozzarella

Also:

2 tablespoons diet Italian dressing

Salt and pepper

Combine all ingredients and toss. Season with salt and pepper to taste.

YIELD: 1 serving

CALORIES: 169

RECIPE #3

HAWAIIAN CHICKEN

INGREDIENTS:

1 whole chicken breast, skinned and boned (7 ounces)

1 teaspoon low-calorie margarine, melted

2 tablespoons pineapple juice

¼ teaspoon dried rosemary

Salt and pepper to taste

1 slice canned pineapple, juice-packed

Paprika

Preheat broiler. Separate chicken breast into halves. Discard fat and membranes. Combine melted margarine, pineapple juice, rosemary, salt, and pepper. Stir to blend.

Place both halves of chicken breast into a shallow broiler pan. Pour above liquid mixture over top of chicken. Broil for 4 minutes about 4 inches below heat source. Turn chicken over and spoon liquid on top. Place pineapple slice on top of one half of chicken breast and continue broiling both halves for another 5 minutes, or until done. Remove from oven and sprinkle with paprika.

Wrap chicken breast without pineapple slice in foil and place in refrigerator for Tuesday's dinner.

YIELD: 2 servings

CALORIES: 215/serving with pineapple slice

179/serving without pineapple slice

RECIPE #4

GRILLED TOMATO

INGREDIENTS:

1 medium (3 inch diameter) tomato

Salt and pepper to taste

1 teaspoon bread crumbs

Dash garlic powder

1 teaspoon minced onion

Pinch dried basil

½ teaspoon vegetable oil

½ teaspoon dried parsley

Preheat broiler. Cut away and discard stem-end slice of tomato and the core. Sprinkle tomato lightly with salt and pepper. Combine bread crumbs, garlic powder, onion, basil, oil, and parsley. Pat mixture over top of tomato, and broil for 6 to 7 minutes, until tomato is heated through and slightly softened.

YIELD: 1 serving

CALORIES: 59

RECIPE #5

CHICKEN CHOWDER

INGREDIENTS:

1½ cups tomato juice or vegetable juice cocktail

3 tablespoons chopped onion

3 tablespoons chopped green pepper

2 tablespoons diced celery

⅓ cup diced potato

¼ teaspoon dried basil

Remaining half of chicken breast from recipe #3, diced

Freshly ground pepper

Combine first five ingredients in a small saucepan. Bring to a boil, reduce heat, and simmer until vegetables are tender, about 10 to 15 minutes. Add basil and diced chicken. Heat thoroughly. Taste, and add seasoning as desired.

YIELD: 1 serving
CALORIES: 205

RECIPE #6

ZESTY SPAGHETTI

INGREDIENTS:

2 ounces (dry weight) spaghetti, cooked
Vegetable cooking spray
½ cup Marinara Sauce (see recipe below)

1 ounce part-skim mozzarella cheese, grated
1 teaspoon grated Parmesan cheese

Preheat oven to 325° F. Cook spaghetti al dente, according to package directions; drain. Treat a single-serving casserole dish with vegetable cooking spray. Add cooked spaghetti to dish and add Marinara Sauce. Stir to coat spaghetti evenly with sauce. Top with grated mozzarella. Bake until cheese bubbles and starts to brown, approximately 10 to 15 minutes. Remove from oven, sprinkle with Parmesan, and serve.

YIELD: 1 serving
CALORIES: 298

MARINARA SAUCE

INGREDIENTS:

12 ounces canned tomato juice

10 ounces canned stewed
  tomatoes

1 teaspoon minced onion

¼ pound fresh mushrooms,
  sliced

½ sweet red pepper, chopped

1 medium green pepper,
  chopped

½ teaspoon dried Italian
  seasoning

Dash garlic powder

Salt and pepper to taste

Combine all ingredients in a heavy saucepan; simmer, uncovered, 45 minutes. (Divide leftover sauce into individual ½ cup serving size freezer containers, freeze. Thaw and use as needed.)

YIELD: approximately 2½ cups

CALORIES: 32 per ½ cup serving

RECIPE #7

STUFFED POTATO

INGREDIENTS:

1 8-ounce baking potato

2 slices packaged ham (25
  calories per slice) cut in
  pieces

½ ounce part-skim mozzarella
  cheese, shredded

½ tablespoon green onion

Prick potato with fork and bake in preheated oven at 400° F. for 1 hour, or until tender. Split top of potato lengthwise. Fluff potato pulp with fork. Place ham pieces and shredded cheese on top, and wrap potato in aluminum foil. Bake another 5 to 7 minutes, until cheese melts. Garnish with green onion.

YIELD: 1 serving
CALORIES: 208

RECIPE #8

GINGER FISH

INGREDIENTS:

4 ounces fillet of flounder (fresh or frozen)
1½ teaspoons honey
1 tablespoon vegetable oil
⅛ teaspoon ground ginger

1 tablespoon lime juice (fresh or bottled)
Salt to taste
Vegetable cooking spray

Thaw fish, if frozen. Place in shallow pan. Combine honey, oil, ginger, lime juice, and salt. Mix well and pour over fish. Cover and chill for several hours, turning fish occasionally.

Preheat broiler. Remove fish from pan, reserving marinade. Spray broiler pan with vegetable cooking spray. Arrange fillet so it is uniform in thickness. Broil 4 inches from heat until fish flakes easily when tested with a fork. Baste often with marinade. (Allow 5 minutes cooking time for each ½ inch of thickness. If fillet is thicker than 1 inch, turn halfway through cooking time.) Brush with marinade just before serving.

YIELD: 1 serving
CALORIES: 161

RECIPE #9

ORANGE CHICKEN

INGREDIENTS:

¾ cup orange juice

½ teaspoon dried rosemary

½ teaspoon dried parsley

4 ounces chicken breast,
   skinned and boned

Mix orange juice and herbs in small ovenproof bowl. Add chicken to bowl and marinate in refrigerator for 2 hours.

Preheat oven to 325° F. Place chicken in oven and bake for 20 to 25 minutes, or until chicken is tender.

YIELD: 1 serving

CALORIES: 198

RECIPE #10

BEEF ORIENTAL

INGREDIENTS:

7 ounces (raw weight) lean
  round steak (¾ inch thick)

1 teaspoon cornstarch

Pinch ground ginger

2 tablespoons low-sodium soy
  sauce

Vegetable cooking spray

1 small green pepper (2¾
  inch diameter), cut into ½
  inch squares

½ cup diced onion

¼ cup sliced carrot

3 tablespoons water

1 small clove garlic, minced

1 tomato (2½ inch diameter),
  cut into 1 inch cubes

Place steak briefly in freezer until firm (makes slicing easier). Slice steak diagonally across the grain into very thin strips—as thin as possible.

Combine cornstarch, ginger, and soy sauce in a small bowl. Add meat and toss to coat each slice. Coat a nonstick skillet with vegetable cooking spray. Heat skillet over medium heat. Add meat and brown quickly, stirring to brown all surfaces. Remove with slotted spoon, and set aside. Add green pepper, onion, carrot, water, and garlic. Cook until carrot and pepper are tender-crisp (5 to 6 minutes). Stir in meat and tomato. Heat thoroughly.

Divide into two portions and freeze one for another meal.

YIELD: 2 servings
CALORIES: 241 per serving

RECIPE #11

SCALLOP DINNER

388 calories   (Optional
   replacement meal for weeks
   3–6)

INGREDIENTS:

6 ounces (raw weight) scallops
2 teaspoons low-calorie
   margarine
Pinch dried basil

Pinch dried tarragon
Salt and freshly ground pepper
Paprika
Lemon wedge

Wash scallops and pat dry. Melt margarine in small skillet and mix with herbs, salt, and pepper. Add scallops to skillet. Stir-fry scallops in herb margarine until done (when they lose their translucency, usually 5 to 8 minutes). Sprinkle with paprika. Serve over rice with fresh lemon wedge.

YIELD: 1 serving
CALORIES: 220

Salad:

2 cups chopped lettuce (18)
¼ cup sliced mushrooms (5)
1 small celery stalk (4 inches
   long), chopped (3)

2 tablespoons grated carrot (6)
2 slices tomato, chopped (14)
1 tablespoon diet Italian
   dressing (6)

Also:

½ cup steamed brown rice
   (116)
Noncaloric beverage

RECIPE #12

PORK CHOP DINNER

387 calories   (Optional
  replacement meal for weeks
  5 and 6)

INGREDIENTS:

1 tablespoon low-calorie
  margarine
1 3-ounce pork chop, no bone
  or fat

¾ cup sliced onion
Salt and pepper to taste

Melt margarine in medium-sized skillet. Brown pork chop for 2 minutes on each side. Add onion, salt, and pepper and cook 4 to 5 minutes more until done.

YIELD: 1 serving
CALORIES: 285

Salad:

2 cups chopped lettuce (18)
¼ cup sliced mushrooms (5)
1 small celery stalk (4 inches
  long), chopped (3)

2 tablespoons grated carrot (6)
2 slices tomato, chopped (14)
1 tablespoon diet Italian dressing (6)

Also:

¾ cup applesauce, sprinkled
with cinnamon and low-calorie
sweetener (50)
Noncaloric beverage

9

▪ SHOPPING LIST ▪

The following shopping list tells you everything one person will need to follow the Makeover Diet menus and recipes for week 1. You simply repeat the food purchases, with slight modifications, for weeks 2, 3, 4, 5, and 6.

Some foods—such as seasonings, packaged goods, and frozen products—will last for many weeks. You may purchase these foods in greater amounts than those listed on a weekly basis. Other foods—such as poultry, beef, and especially fish—may not remain fresh for even a few days unless you freeze them. Always keep the perishability of the food in mind when you are using the shopping list.

Quantities needed for items marked with a box (▪) will depend on your individual selections for Basic Breakfasts and Basic Lunches. Review your choices and adjust the shopping list accordingly. You may vary these selections from week to week.

HAVE ON HAND

Staples
- beverages, noncaloric (water, coffee, tea, diet soft drinks)
- bouillon, low-sodium
  bread, reduced-calorie (40 calories per slice)
  bread crumbs, dried
  brown rice, 1 cup steamed
  cereal (110 calories per 1-ounce serving), choose from:
  Nabisco Shredded Wheat
  Kellogg's Frosted Mini Wheats
  Kellogg's NutriGrain wheat or corn
  Post Grape Nuts
  Ralston Purina Almond Delight
  Ralston Purina Sun Flakes Crispy Wheat & Rice
  oatmeal
  cheese, part-skim mozzarella
  cheese, Parmesan (grated)
  cinnamon
  cornstarch
  diet Italian dressing (6 calories per tablespoon)
  graham crackers
  dried basil
  honey
- low-calorie sweetener
  low-sodium soy sauce
  margarine, low-calorie (50 calories per tablespoon)
  mayonnaise, low-calorie (40 calories per tablespoon)

milk, skim
pepper, fresh ground
raisins
- saltines
spaghetti, 2 ounces dry
- vanilla
vegetable cooking oil
vegetable cooking spray
- wheat germ

FRUITS, VEGETABLES, JUICES

acorn squash (4 inch diameter)
- applesauce, unsweetened (⅔ cup per serving)
banana, medium (8¾ inches long)
- bananas, large (9¾ inches long)
- blueberries, fresh or frozen (⅔ cup per serving)
broccoli, chopped, 1 cup
- cantaloupe, fresh or frozen (⅔ cup per serving)
carrots
celery
corn on the cob (5 inches long), fresh or frozen, 2 ears
- cucumber(s)
green beans, French-style, fresh or frozen, 2 cups
- green onion
green peppers, 3
- lemon, fresh, 1 large
lettuce, 1 large head
lime, fresh, 1 large
- mushrooms, fresh, 1 pound
onion, red, 1 small
onion, white, 1 small

orange juice, unsweetened, 34 ounces

peach, medium (6 ounces, 2¾ inch diameter), 2,
   or canned pears, juice-packed, 1 cup

pineapple, canned, juice-packed, 2 slices

potato, 8-ounce baking

potatoes, small (2½ inch diameter, 4½ ounces), 2

red pepper, sweet, 1 small

spinach, fresh leaves, 2 cups

■ strawberries (fresh or frozen without sugar)

tomato juice, canned, 12 ounces

tomatoes, canned stewed, 10 ounces

tomatoes, fresh, medium (3 inch diameter), 3; small (2½ inch
   diameter), 1

vegetable juice cocktail, 24 ounces

HERBS, SPICES, SEASONINGS

basil, dried

cinnamon

garlic clove

garlic powder

ginger, ground

Italian seasoning, dried

paprika

parsley, dried

pepper

rosemary, dried

salt

MEAT, FISH, POULTRY

- chicken, roasted, skinned (2 ounces per serving)
  chicken breasts, whole (12 ounces raw weight)
  flounder fillet, fresh or frozen, 4 ounces
- ham, baked, or packaged, sliced ham (trimmed of excess fat) (1½ ounces per serving)
- roast beef, lean sliced (2 ounces per serving)
- round steak, lean, 7 ounces raw weight, ¾-inch thick
- tuna, water-packed (½ 6½ ounce can per serving)
- turkey, roasted, skinned (2 ounces per serving)

DAIRY PRODUCTS

- cheese, Swiss or Monterey Jack (1 ounce per serving)
  ice milk (100 calories per ½ cup serving), 1 cup

PART III

▪EXERCISING▪

10

•THE KEYS TO PRODUCTIVE EXERCISE: HIGH INTENSITY AND SUPER SLOW •

Dieting—without the right type of exercising—is a very big mistake.

Yes, it's possible to lose weight with diet alone. But research shows that from 25 to 90 percent of the weight loss comes not from body fat, but from the muscles, organs, and fluids. Loss of proteins and fluids from these vital cells is not healthy. Furthermore, dieting without exercising dramatically reduces your metabolic rate and makes keeping the lost weight off next to impossible.

Remember, one of the goals of the Fat-to-Muscle Makeover is to make sure that the weight you lose on this program is FAT. The only way to be sure that your weight loss is truly fat is to combine a descending-calorie diet with high-intensity exercise.

High-intensity exercise stimulates your muscles to become larger and stronger. Stimulating your muscles at the same time you reduce dietary calories assures that fluids will remain in your lean body mass. Research reveals that your body can lose fat and gain muscle simultaneously. As you have noticed in the statistics that accompany the before-and-after photographs in Part I, that is exactly what the Six-Week Fat-to-Muscle Makeover helps you do.

HIGH-INTENSITY EXERCISE DEFINED

High intensity means performing an exercise to the point of momentary muscular fatigue; a point reached when it is temporarily impossible to achieve another repetition properly.

For high-intensity exercise to be consistently effective, it must involve the lifting and lowering of progressively heavier weights. Weights in the form of adjustable dumbbells, barbells, Nautilus machines, or other selectorized weight machines must be used in this form of exercise.

High-intensity training is not an easy form of exercise. It's difficult, demanding, and brutally hard. In fact, at the start of many of my research projects, I often tell the women, "This whole experience is going to be treated like a Vince Lombardi Green Bay Packer football camp. If you're not serious about losing fat and keeping it off, don't get involved with this program."

I feel the same way about this book, especially the high-intensity exercise part of it.

Naturally, a few women will be turned off by my approach. But such types usually do not have the discipline and patience to stick with anything demanding for very long. They are better off *not* getting involved. The women who respond best to the high-intensity challenge are usually the ones who are tired of quick-and-easy weight-loss schemes that produce only short-term effects.

The problem with so many diet/exercise programs is that the type of exercise prescribed is too low in intensity to build muscle. Dance exercise, swimming laps, jogging, walking, and cycling are all ways to improve your cardiovascular fitness, and they do burn calories. But they do not stimulate your muscles to grow larger and stronger. The only way to accomplish growth stimulation is with high-intensity exercise. Your muscles respond to this all-out effort by growing larger. And remember, the more muscle you have, the more calories you can take in each day without gaining fat.

A typical high-intensity workout lasts only 20 minutes. But for that 20 minutes you must be willing to give each exercise your best effort. You must be willing to make your workout hard, brief, and challenging if you want to get the best possible results.

Maximum results in the most efficient manner. That's the goal of high-intensity exercise, as well as the overall theme of the Fat-to-Muscle Makeover.

SPEED OF MOVEMENT

Of equal importance to the intensity of the exercise is your speed of lifting and lowering the weight on each repetition. Since 1982 two of my associates, Ken and Brenda Hutchins, and I have been researching the effects of performing each repetition of an exercise very slowly. This form of exercise, which we've appropriately named super slow, requires lifting the weight in 10 seconds and lowering it in 4 seconds.

We've discovered that there are three major advantages that super slow has over traditional, faster styles of performing repetitions.

1 ▪ *Super slow supplies more thorough muscle-fiber involvement.* When you move slowly during a repetition, you significantly reduce the momentum that normally occurs. As a result you activate parts of the muscle that are not usually brought into play.

2 ▪ *Super slow is safer.* Since you are now lifting the weight in a smooth, controlled fashion, there are no quick jerks and drops. Thus, the force on the muscle remains steady and much safer than traditional fast, jerky styles of lifting.

3 ▪ *Super slow produces better strength-building results.* How much better? Studies show that compared to the normal way of performing a repetition (2 seconds up and 4 seconds down), women doing super slow (10 seconds up and 4 seconds down) received 59 percent better gains.

So super-slow training, compared to the normal way of lifting and lowering weight, is much more productive at building strength. It's the ideal form of exercise to combine with a descending-calorie diet.

THE FINER POINTS OF SUPER SLOW

In super-slow training you lift the weight in approximately 10 seconds, then lower it to the beginning position in 4 seconds. Using the leg extension exercise as an example should help make the mechanics of super slow clear.

Place a light amount of weight on a standard leg extension machine. Sit in the machine with your ankles behind the roller pads. Your knees should be bent. Instead of lifting the weight suddenly by straightening your legs, do the following:

- Try to barely start to move the resistance, maybe by only a perceptible ⅛ inch.
- Proceed slowly and smoothly once you start moving.
- Continue to straighten your legs and arrive at the fully extended position at about the 10-second mark. Initially, someone with a stopwatch should help you with the training.
- Pause in the extended position.

- Ease out of the top position gradually. Smoothly increase speed, but still move slowly, and return to the starting position in about 4 seconds.
- Feel the weight stack touch, but do not let the slack out of the chain, or rest. You want to touch, then barely move again in the upward direction.
- Concentrate on keeping the movement arm traveling at a near-constant speed. Do not alternately try to stop and heave into the resistance.
- Keep the lifting slow, but steady—and the lowering smooth.
- Stop after you've experienced four or five correct repetitions.

Even with a light weight you should begin to feel a burning sensation in your frontal thighs. Do not be alarmed. The burning is perfectly natural and an indication that the involved muscle fibers are being thoroughly worked.

Once you get the hang of super slow, you should select a resistance that will permit you to perform between four and eight repetitions. When you can do eight or more repetitions in good form, that is the signal to increase your resistance in the exercise by approximately 5 percent at your next workout.

BASIC SUPER-SLOW GUIDELINES

Super slow can be employed with almost any type of weight-training equipment: Nautilus, barbells, dumbbells, or even using your own body weight. The following guidelines apply no matter what equipment you use.

1 ▪ Perform three to five exercises for your lower body and five to seven exercises for your upper body, and no more than ten exercises in any workout.

2 ▪ Train no more than three, nonconsecutive days per week. High-intensity exercise necessitates a recovery period of at least 48 hours. Your body gets stronger during rest, not during exercise.

3 ▪ Select a resistance for each exercise that allows the performance of between four and eight super-slow repetitions.

    a   Begin with a weight with which you can comfortably do four repetitions.

    b   Stay with that weight until eight or more strict repetitions are performed. In the following workout, increase the resistance by 5 percent.

    c   Attempt constantly to increase the number of repetitions or the amount of weight, or both. But do not sacrifice form in an attempt to produce repetition and resistance improvements.

4 ▪ Concentrate on each repetition by lifting the weight slowly in 10 seconds, and lowering it smoothly in 4 seconds.

5 ▪ Move slower, never faster, if in doubt about the speed of movement.

6 ▪ Relax body parts that are not involved in each exercise. Pay special attention to relaxing your face, neck, and hand muscles.

7 ▪ Breathe normally. Try not to hold your breath during any repetition.

8 ▪ Keep accurate records—date, resistance, repetitions, and overall training time—of each workout.

THE NAUTILUS ADVANTAGE

I am the Director of Research for Nautilus Sports/Medical Industries and a firm believer in the effectiveness of the Nautilus equipment. It's safer and easier to use than dumbbells or barbells, and, unlike many other brands of weight machines, Nautilus machines are designed to work specific muscle groups through a full range of movement.

A beginner can learn to use the Nautilus equipment safely and effectively in two or three workouts. Availability is usually not a problem, since there are more than 5,000 specialized Nautilus facilities in the United States. Organizations such as YMCAs, universities and colleges, recreation centers, government agencies, and the armed forces also may provide access to Nautilus equipment.

It's important, however, to mention that even if you don't have access to Nautilus equipment, you can still do the Makeover program. With ingenuity and practice, you can use other brands of weight machines or free weights to duplicate the Nautilus exercises. In fact, Chapter 12 shows you how to do a productive workout with dumbbells and calisthenic exercises.

But for now let's concentrate on how to get maximum results from the use of Nautilus equipment, which is the subject of the next chapter.

11

·MAKEOVER NAUTILUS ROUTINES·

Each woman who went through the Six-Week Fat-to-Muscle Makeover under my supervision in Florida in 1986 and 1987 added almost 4 pounds of figure-shaping muscle. Remember, larger and stronger muscles are a primary factor in getting the lean, firm body that you've always wanted. And building more shapely muscles is the secret to permanent fat loss.

The super-slow, high-intensity Nautilus program stresses three nonconsecutive day, 20-minute workouts per week. You perform only six exercises during weeks 1 and 2. Increase to eight exercises during weeks 3 and 4. The final two weeks you employ a maximum of ten exercises.

YOU'LL GET STRONGER

You'll be excited over how much stronger you become. As was noted in Chapter 10, when you can perform eight super-slow repetitions in good form, increase the weight by 5 percent at your next workout. Always strive to increase the amount of resistance or number of repetitions—or both—at each successive workout.

You will add two new exercises every two weeks, while increasing weight and/or repetitions in the other exercises. Never let your workout get easier: move up in resistance (weight) or repetitions. This is the concept of progressive-resistance exercise.

And it works.

The women in DeLand were given a sixth-week workout with the weights set back to their starting levels—and they couldn't believe the difference. What had seemed to be a maximum effort weeks before had become easy.

Six weeks of efficient, hard and brief workouts does wonders for your physical conditioning, as well as your appearance.

A 56-year-old trainee brought her 37-year-old daughter to one of her workouts late in the DeLand program. After mom had gone through her usual workout, the daughter tried a couple of exercises. To mom's delight, the weights had to be reduced—her daughter couldn't handle as much resistance.

In another instance a visiting husband had difficulty matching his wife's output on the lower body exercises.

TEST STRENGTH BEFORE AND AFTER

If you're using Nautilus equipment, measure your starting strength level on the leg extension and leg curl (lower body), the pullover and abdominal (upper body).

Through trial and error during the first week, determine the maximum weight you can lift six times with good form. Add the weight of leg extension and leg curl and divide by two. This is your starting lower body strength.

Add the weight of pullover and abdominal and divide by two to determine your starting upper body strength.

Repeat this procedure during the sixth week. Expect an increase of about 30 percent in the lower body and 30 percent in the upper body.

WORKOUT ROUTINE

What exercises should you do?

Here are the exact Nautilus routines that the Florida women followed on the Makeover program. They are also the best routines for you to use.

If you do not have access to the exact Nautilus machines that are listed in the routines below, do not fret. You can easily substitute other machines in place of them. For example, you can substitute the Decline Press for the Bench Press, the 10-Degree Chest for the Arm Cross, or the Duo Hip and Back for the Hip Abduction. Be sure to check with your local Nautilus instructor for assistance in performing on any substituted machines.

Madelaine Wildman, who is featured in Chapter 1, demonstrates the Nautilus exercises that helped transform her figure from fatness to fitness—in only six weeks!

MAKEOVER NAUTILUS ROUTINES

WEEKS 1 AND 2	WEEKS 3 AND 4	WEEKS 5 AND 6
1. Leg Extension	1. Leg Extension	1. Leg Extension
2. Leg Curl	2. Leg Curl	2. Leg Curl
3. Hip Adduction	3. Hip Abduction*	3. Hip Abduction
4. Pullover	4. Hip Adduction	4. Hip Adduction
5. Bench Press	5. Pullover	5. Calf Raise on Multi-Exercise*
6. Abdominal	6. Bench Press	6. Pullover
	7. Multi-Biceps*	7. Arm Cross*
	8. Abdominal	8. Bench Press
		9. Multi-Biceps
*Indicates new exercise		10. Abdominal

DISCIPLINE AND PATIENCE

The Nautilus routines helped Madelaine Wildman lose 18¼ pounds of body fat, 3 inches from her waist, and 6 inches from her thighs.

Similar reshaping of your own body can take place—if you apply the necessary discipline and patience.

Get involved now!

Leg extension, contracted position.

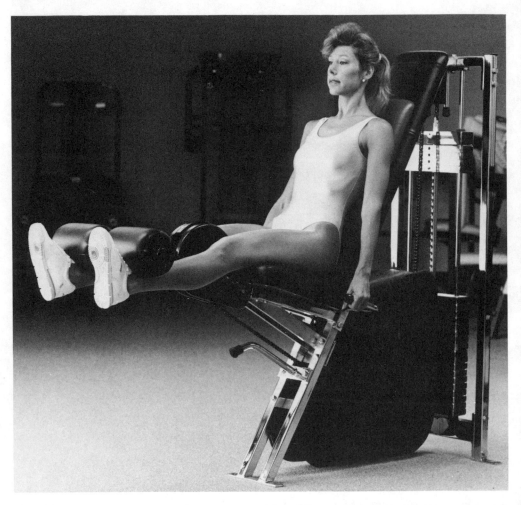

Leg extension for front of thighs: Sit in machine. Place ankles behind roller pads, with knees snug against seat bottom and torso against seat back. Some women may require a long pad to be placed between their buttocks and the seat back. If machine has a seat belt, fasten it across hips. Grasp handles lightly. Straighten both legs in 10 seconds. Pause. Lower legs in 4 seconds. Repeat for maximum repetitions.

Leg curl, contracted position.

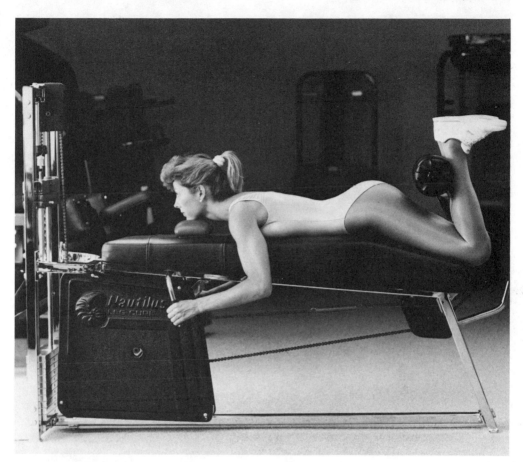

Leg curl for back of thighs: Lie facedown on machine. Place feet under roller pads with knees just over edge of bench. Grasp handles to keep body from moving. Curl both legs in 10 seconds and try to touch heels to buttocks. Pause. Uncurl in 4 seconds. Repeat for maximum repetitions.

Hip adduction, starting position.

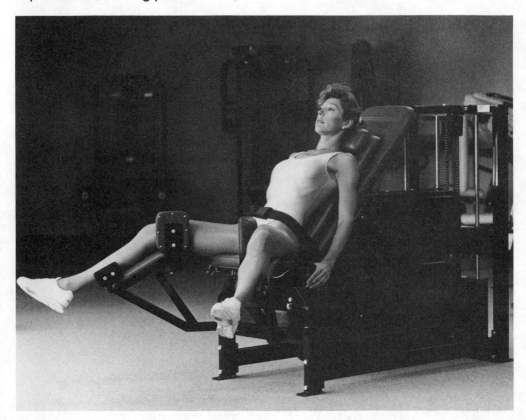

Hip adduction for inner thighs: Adjust lever on right side of machine for range of movement. Sit in machine and place knees and ankles on movement arms in a spread-legged position. Most women will require an additional back pad and/or head pad for support. Fasten seat belt. Pull knees and thighs together in 10 seconds. Pause in knees-together position. Return to stretched position in 4 seconds. Repeat for maximum repetitions.

Pullover, midrange position.

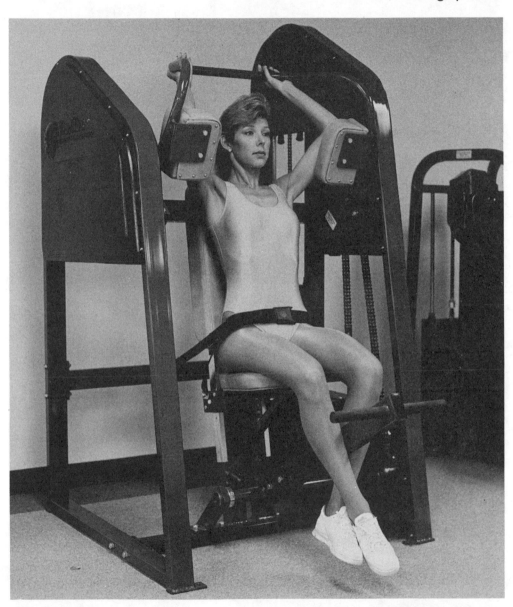

Pullover for back: Adjust seat so shoulder joints are in line with axes of rotation of movement arm. Assume erect position and fasten seat belt. Leg press foot pedal until elbow pads are about chin level. Place elbows on pads. Remove legs from pedal and rotate elbows back for comfortable stretch. This is the starting position. Rotate elbows forward and down in 10 seconds. Pause with bar on midsection. Return to stretched position in 4 seconds. Repeat for maximum repetitions.

Bench press, extended position.

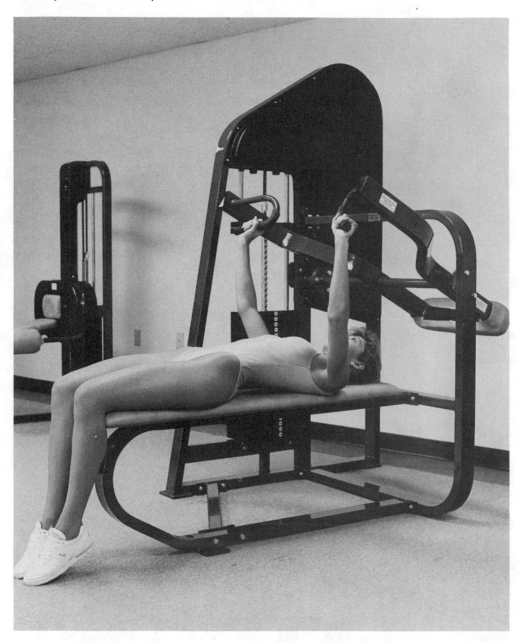

Bench press for shoulders, chest, and arms: Lie on back. Hand grips should be beside chest. Place hands on grips. Stabilize feet and legs. Press handles and movement arm over chest in 10 seconds. Do not grip handles excessively hard. Lower hands in 4 seconds to starting position. Repeat for maximum repetitions.

Abdominal, contracted position.

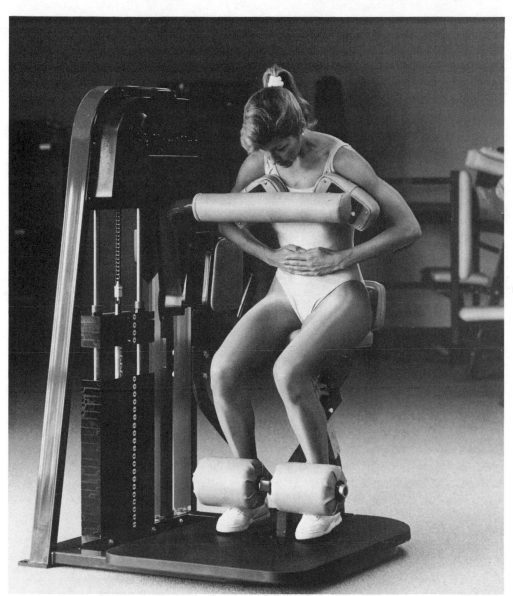

Abdominal for waist: Sit in machine with swivel pads in front of chest. Move swivel pads to comfortable position on chest. Adjust seat until axis of rotation of movement arm is parallel to navel. Women with thin hips may need a small pad placed between seat back and buttocks. Hook feet under bottom roller pads. Place hands across waist. Move chest toward hips in 10 seconds. Pause. Return to starting position in 4 seconds. Do not arch lower back; keep it rounded. Repeat for maximum repetitions.

Hip abduction, starting position.

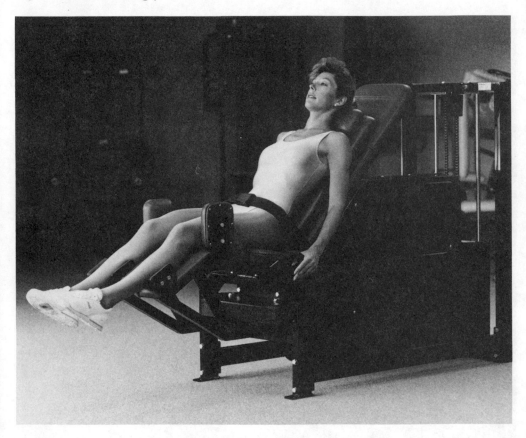

Hip abduction for outer hips and thighs: Sit in machine and place legs on movement arms. Most women will require an additional back pad and/or head pad for support. Fasten seat belt. Push knees and thighs apart to widest position in 10 seconds. Pause. Return to knees-together position in 4 seconds. Repeat for maximum repetitions.

Multi-biceps, starting position.

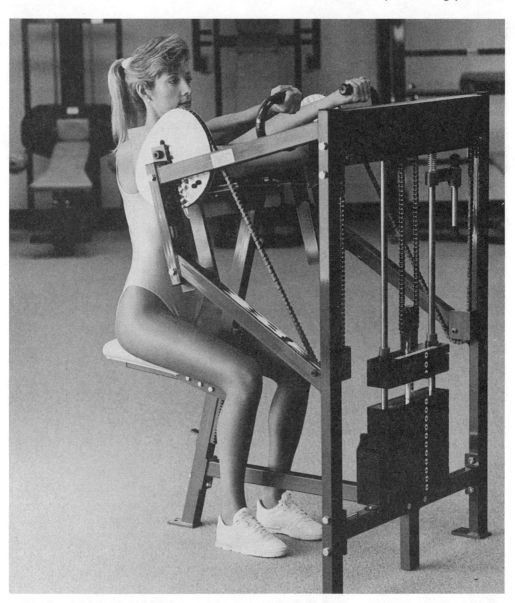

Multi-biceps for upper arms: Stand and place elbows in line with axes of movement arms. Grasp handles lightly. Bend arms to 90 degrees and be seated. Lower hands until elbows are straight. Shoulders should be slightly lower than elbows. If not, relax arms and readjust seat. Curl both arms in 10 seconds. Thumbs should almost touch shoulders in contracted position. Pause. Lower arms to starting position in 4 seconds. Repeat for maximum repetitions.

Calf raise on Multi-Exercise machine, stretched position.

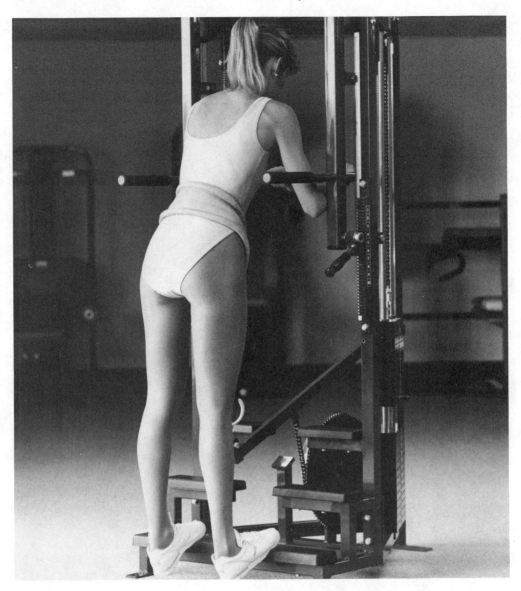

Calf raise for back calves: Attach steel ring of padded belt to hook snap on movement arm of Multi-Exercise machine. Grasp padded belt, place both feet through it while facing machine, and kneel on first step. Move belt around hips and stand up. Adjust belt to comfortable position. Place balls of feet on first step and hands on front of carriage. Lock knees and keep locked throughout movement. Elevate heels in 10 seconds and try to stand on tiptoes. Pause in highest position. Lower heels in 4 seconds. Stretch. Repeat for maximum repetitions.

Arm cross on Women's, Men's, or Double Chest Machine, contracted position.

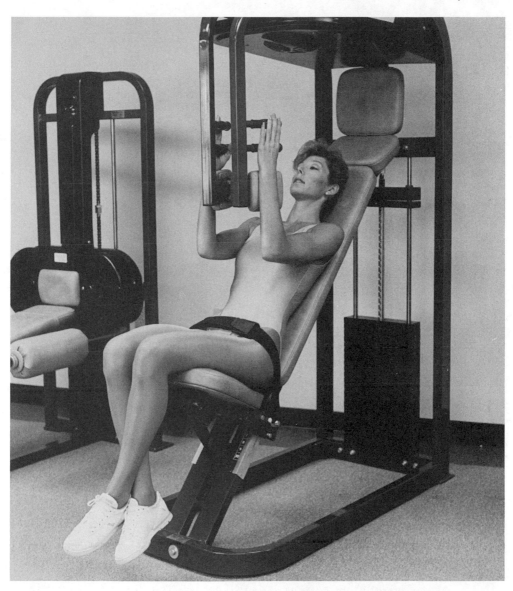

Arm cross for chest: Adjust seat until shoulders, with elbows held together, are directly under the overhead axes of the movement arms. Some women may require an extra back pad to put their shoulders in proper alignment. Fasten seat belt. Place forearms behind and firmly against pads of movement arms. Grasp handles lightly with thumbs around handles. Keep head and back against seat back. Push with forearms and try to touch elbows together in front of chest in 10 seconds. Pause in contracted position. Lower resistance in 4 seconds to stretched position. Repeat for maximum repetitions.

12

▪MAKEOVER DUMBBELL ROUTINES▪

If it is not possible for you to train on Nautilus equipment, you can still get a result-producing workout using dumbbells and a few calisthenic-type exercises.

In fact, one group of women in Orlando went through the six-week program and performed all their exercises using conventional dumbbells and their own body weight. They applied the same super-slow, high-intensity guidelines that were described in Chapter 10.

The overall results were almost as good as those of the Nautilus-trained women. Each woman in the dumbbell group gained 3.11 pounds of muscle, compared to 3.87 for the Nautilus group. In other words, training with dumbbells produced approximately 80 percent of the results that Nautilus did, at least for six weeks.

So even if you cannot use Nautilus equipment, you can still get dramatic body-shaping results from exercising with dumbbells. The secret is not so much in the equipment—but in *how you use* what you have available to you.

The best way to use Nautilus, barbells, dumbbells, and calisthenics is in the super-slow, high-intensity manner.

For the six-week dumbbell routines you'll need a pair of adjustable dumbbells and some small weight plates in increments of 1¼, 2½, and 5 pounds. Or you may choose to purchase pairs of solid dumbbells that range from 5 to 20 pounds each. Or in a bind you can use two 1-gallon plastic bottles of water as your adjustable dumbbells. (Note: A gallon of water weighs approximately 8 pounds.)

Use enough resistance on the recommended dumbbell exercises to perform one set of from four to eight super-slow repetitions. When you can do eight or more repetitions in correct form, increase the combined weight of both dumbbells by approximately 5 percent at your next workout. Remember, each workout should be hard, brief, and repeated three times per week.

The photos on the following pages showing dumbbell exercises were taken of Lysa Parker after she completed the Fat-to-Muscle Makeover. Lysa's story is told in Chapter 1.

HARDER AND SLOWER

The dumbbell routines can be used in the privacy of your home or even adapted for use in a hotel room as you travel. And as stated previously, they can be very productive—especially if you look for little ways to make the movements harder, rather than easier. Super-slow movements are a way to do just that.

LISTED BELOW ARE THE DUMBBELL ROUTINES

MAKEOVER DUMBBELL ROUTINES

WEEKS 1 AND 2	WEEKS 3 AND 4	WEEKS 5 AND 6
1. Squat with dumbbells	1. Squat with dumbbells	1. Squat with dumbbells
2. Pullover with dumbbell	2. Calf raise on one leg*	2. Calf raise on one leg
3. Lateral raise with dumbbells	3. Pullover with dumbbell	3. Wide-stance squat*
4. Trunk curl	4. Lateral raise with dumbbells	4. Pullover with dumbbell
5. Biceps curl with dumbbells	5. Trunk curl	5. Lateral raise with dumbbells
6. Push-up	6. Biceps curl with dumbbells	6. Trunk curl
	7. Upright rowing with dumbbells*	7. Triceps extension with dumbbell*
	8. Push-up	8. Biceps curl with dumbbells
		9. Upright rowing with dumbbells
*Indicates new exercise		10. Push-up

Squat with dumbbells, bottom position

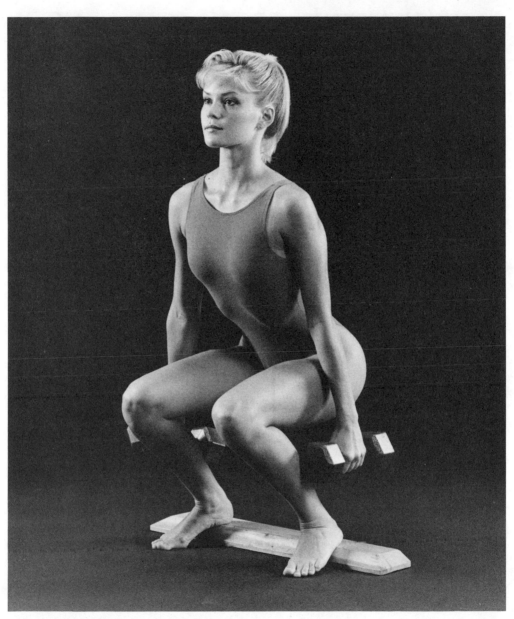

Squat with dumbbells for hips and thighs: Put a small 2-by-6-inch board on the floor. Grasp a dumbbell in each hand, stand erect, and place heels shoulder-width apart on board. Lower body in 4 seconds by bending hips and knees. Do not relax or bounce at the bottom. Return to an almost-erect position in 10 seconds. Do not quite straighten knees. This makes the exercise more demanding. Repeat for maximum repetitions.

Pullover with dumbell, starting position.

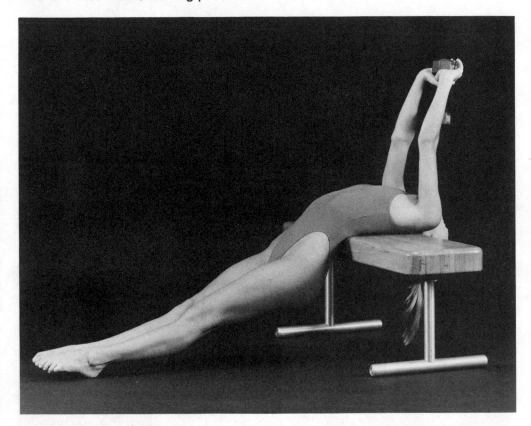

Pullover with dumbbell for back: Lie crossways on sturdy bench with back on bench and head and hips off bench. With both hands, hold one end of a light dumbbell over chest, arms straight. While keeping arms straight, lower dumbbell in 4 seconds behind head toward floor. Stretch in bottom position. Lift dumbbell back over chest in 10 seconds. Repeat for maximum repetitions.

Lateral raise with dumbbells, contracted position.

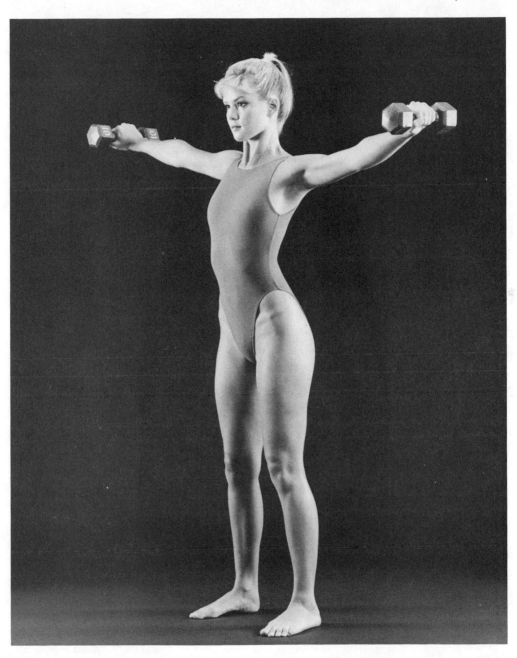

Lateral raise with dumbbells for shoulders: Stand erect, arms at sides, with a dumbbell in each hand. Keep arms straight. Raise dumbbells to shoulder height in 10 seconds. Pause. Lower smoothly in 4 seconds. Repeat for maximum repetitions.

Trunk curl, midrange position.

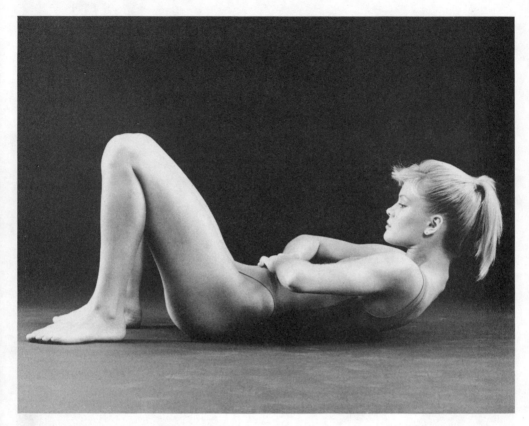

Trunk curl for waist: Lie face up on floor with hands across waist. Bring heels close to buttocks and spread knees. Try lifting shoulders and back off floor as high as possible, and hold in highest position for 10 seconds. Only one-third of a standard sit-up can be performed in this position. Lower shoulders and back to floor in 4 seconds. Repeat for maximum repetitions.

Biceps curl with dumbbells, midrange position.

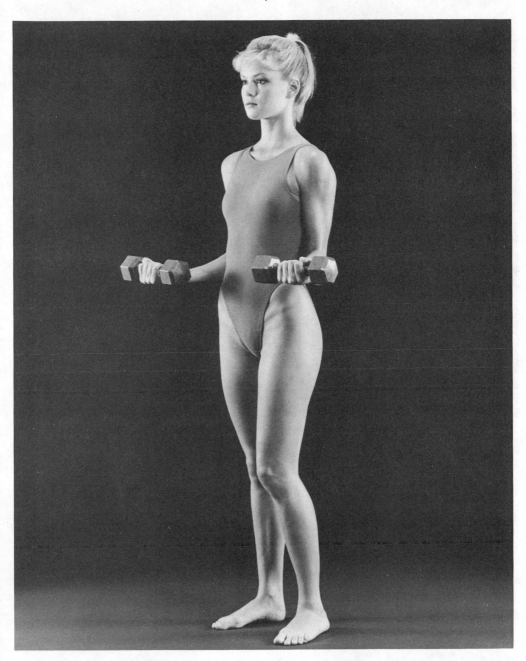

Biceps curl with dumbbells for front of upper arms: Stand erect with a dumbbell in each hand. Stabilize elbows by sides. Curl dumbbells together to shoulder height in 10 seconds. Repeat for maximum repetitions.

Push-up, starting position.

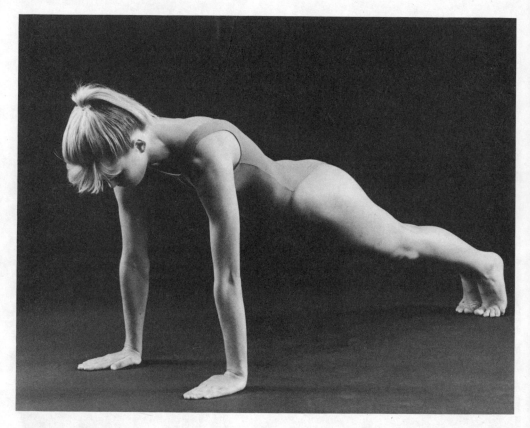

Push-up for chest, shoulders, and upper arms: This is the only exercise you'll do in a lowering-only manner. Assume a standard push-up position on toes and hands with body stiff. Lower body to floor by bending arms in 10 seconds. Do not try to push yourself up to top position. When you reach the floor, bend knees, straighten arms, get back on toes, and stiffen body once again. Perform another slow lowering in 10 seconds. Repeat for at least four repetitions. If you cannot do at least four repetitions, perform the push-up on your knees instead of your toes.

One-legged calf raise, contracted position.

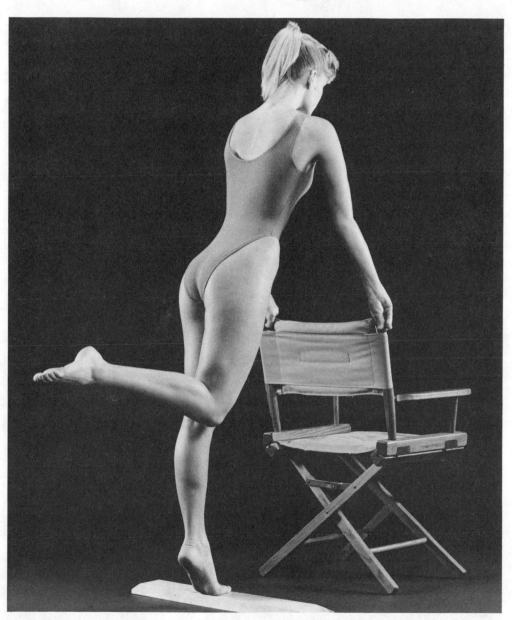

One-legged calf raise with body weight for calves: Place ball of left foot on edge of 2-by-6-inch board or a stair step. Lock left knee and suspend other foot. Balance body by holding onto a chair or stair rail. Raise left heel slowly, in 10 seconds, as high as possible and try to stand on tiptoes. Lower smoothly to deep stretch in 4 seconds. Repeat for maximum repetitions. Follow same procedure for right calf.

Upright rowing with dumbbells, contracted position.

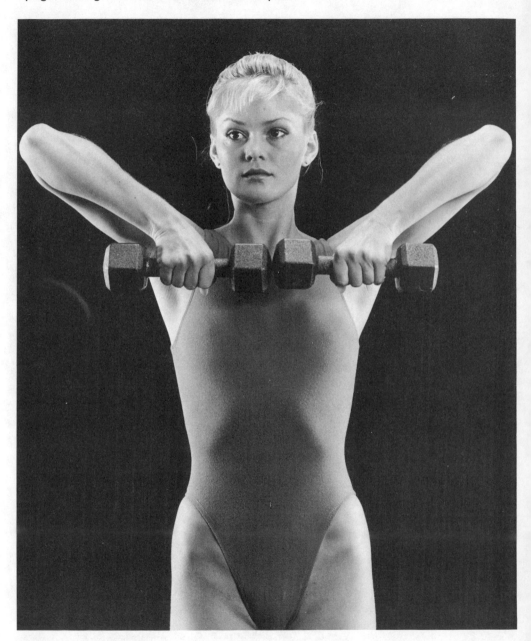

Upright rowing with dumbbells for shoulders: Stand erect with a dumbbell in each hand. Hold dumbbells end-to-end with overhand grip. Raise dumbbells to neck by bending elbows in 10 seconds. Keep elbows higher than dumbbells. Lower dumbbells in 4 seconds, until arms are straight. Repeat for maximum repetitions.

Wide-stance squat, midrange position.

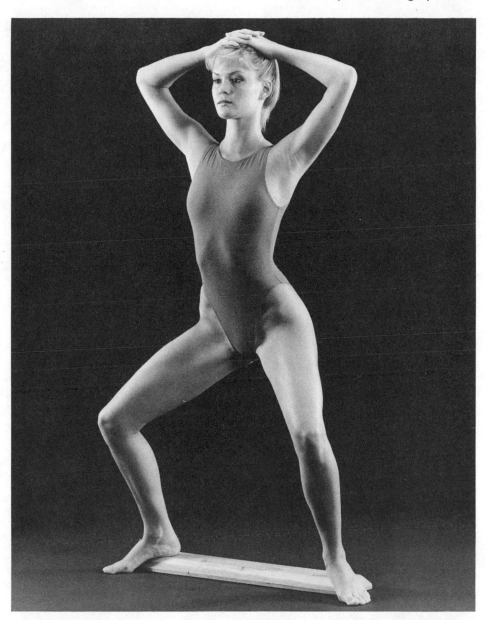

Wide-stance squat for inner thighs: Put a 2-by-6-inch board on the floor. Position heels approximately 24 to 30 inches apart on board. Place hands on head. Lower body by bending hips and knees in 4 seconds. Do not stop or bounce in and out of bottom position. Return to almost-erect position in 10 seconds. Immediately, but smoothly, start lowering again. Repeat for maximum repetitions.

Triceps extension with dumbbell, midrange position.

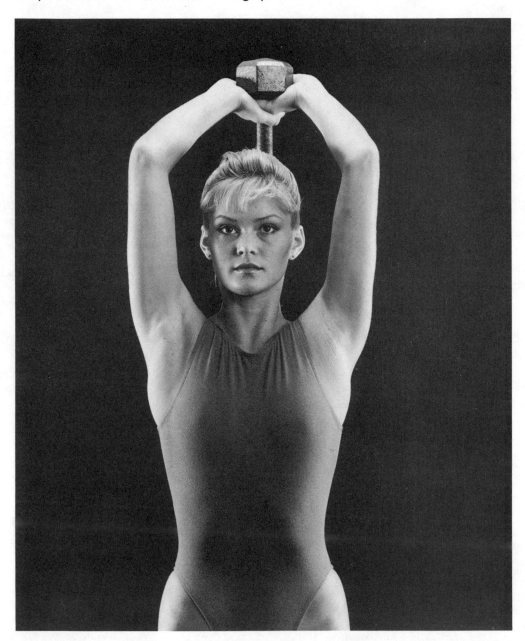

Triceps extension with dumbbell for back of upper arms: With both hands, hold one end of a dumbbell and press it over head. Keep elbows by ears. Lower dumbbell behind head in 4 seconds. Do not move elbows. Raise dumbbell to top position in 10 seconds. Repeat for maximum repetitions.

PART IV

▪ MAINTAINING ▪

13
▪IMPROVING RESULTS AND LONG-TERM MAINTENANCE▪

Make lifetime habits of regular exercise and a sensible plan of calorie intake management. Doing so will assure you your best appearance, and heighten your level of vim and vigor.

That is certainly what it did for Cathe Haigwood, 40, of Orlando.

Said Cathe, "The exercise gives me more satisfaction than I can say because I know I am doing something healthful to make myself stay younger, and to keep my back and neck free from pain. I can tell a difference in my mental attitude."

This chapter discusses how to improve your results by continuing to diet and exercise, and then addresses long-term maintenance.

IMPROVING RESULTS

The key to improving your results is to continue with the same descending-calorie diet and progressive-exercise program for another six weeks. In fact, many of the women in my Florida research did just that.

Two women featured in this chapter, Cathy Allinson, 37, of DeLand, and Trish White, 24, of Orlando, achieved outstanding results in back-to-back Six-Week Fat-to-Muscle Makeovers. In fact, both Cathy and Trish did better during their second session than the first!

You can do the same. Simply turn back to Chapter 5 and follow the 1,200-calorie-a-day menus from weeks 1 and 2. Weeks 3, 4, 5, and 6 are repeated in the same manner.

If you feel that you are familiar enough with basic food groups, servings, calorie counting, and food substitution, you may want to design some of your own meals. Great! Just make sure you keep your daily calories at the appropriate level.

Perhaps you're wondering about going from 1,000 calories a day in week 6, up to 1,200 calories a day in week 7. Won't the rise in calories cause you to regain some of the lost fat?

Actually this down-up-down calorie plan is more effective in producing fat loss than simply sticking to the same number of calories each day, week, and month. It is more result producing for three reasons:

1 ▪ Such a diet provides you with needed variety.
2 ▪ A certain irregularity exists that seems to benefit your body's fat-burning process. Just when your body becomes adjusted to a certain level of energy, the calories go down or up.
3 ▪ When your calories go up, so does your energy level. Such an increase in energy level may be just the motivation you need to exercise harder and thus stimulate additional muscle growth.

CATHY ALLINSON, AGE 37

"THE FIRST SIX WEEKS PROVED TO ME THAT THE PROGRAM WORKED. I HAD A GREAT DEAL OF CONFIDENCE ENTERING THE SECOND SIX WEEKS, AND I WAS ELATED THAT MY FAT LOSS WAS EVEN BETTER."

Lost 27¼ pounds of fat and trimmed 2½ inches off her waist, 3⅝ inches off her hips, 6⅜ inches off her thighs in *twelve* weeks!

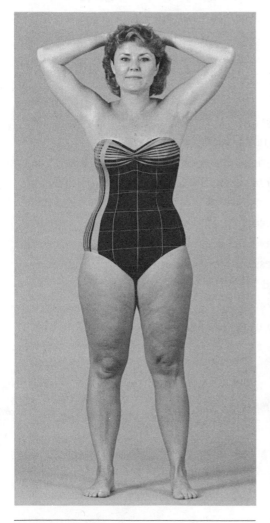

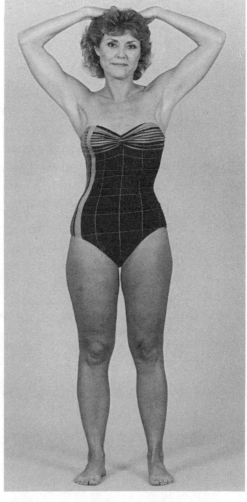

BEFORE
Six-Week Fat-to-Muscle Makeover.

AFTER
Six-Week Fat-to-Muscle Makeover.

EXERCISE ROUTINES

Your three-times-per-week exercise routines—whether with Nautilus or dumbbells—should remain at one set of ten exercises. Continue to follow the guidelines in Chapter 10. You definitely want to keep adding to your weights and repetitions.

How much should you improve each week? Our Florida women improved an average of 5 percent per week for the first six weeks. That's a 30 percent improvement in strength in six weeks, which is very significant. A 30 percent improvement in lower and upper body strength equates to a muscle mass gain of almost 4 pounds.

And please do not worry that the super-slow, high-intensity exercise is going to turn you into a muscular hulk. This will not happen, not even after dozens of years of training.

Building unusually large muscles requires two factors. First, the individual must have long muscle bellies and short tendon attachments. Second, an adequate amount of male hormones, particularly testosterone, must be present in the bloodstream. Women seldom have long muscle bellies; in fact, this is even rare among men. And women on the average have less than one one-hundredth the amount of testosterone in their blood than do men.

If you ever feel you are becoming too muscular, you can reduce your exercising and the extra muscle will diminish. Atrophy is easy to achieve.

LONG-TERM MAINTENANCE: DIETING

Once you reach your goal—whether it takes six weeks, twelve weeks, or even eighteen weeks—a long-term maintenance program becomes not only necessary, but of ultimate importance!

Your goal is now to maintain your present body weight, or more precisely: *your present muscle-fat ratio.* And you maintain your present muscle-fat ratio with *proper diet* and *proper exercise.*

On your maintenance diet, you must still be conscious of calories. Generally speaking, an average lean, fit woman requires from 1,400 to 2,100 calories a day to maintain her ideal muscle-fat ratio.

Once you are satisfied with your body, you will probably fall within this maintenance calorie range. There is no simple way, however, to determine in advance how many calories you will need to maintain your weight. The only way is through trial and error.

Figuring out your maintenance calorie level is done by gradually adding calories from the four basic food groups to the 1,200-calorie-a-day diet (see page 48). For example, you try a certain level—say 1,500 calories a day—for two weeks. Careful weighings show that you are still losing fat. So you raise your calories to 1,700 a day for another two weeks and your weight stabilizes. Now you know you have reached the upper limit of your maintenance caloric level.

Of course all this figuring assumes that your activity and exercise habits remain consistent, which brings us to the topic of maintenance exercising.

LONG-TERM MAINTENANCE: EXERCISING

You must continue to exercise your newly built muscles or they will atrophy, or shrink, with disuse. Don't allow this wasting away to happen to your lean, muscular body. Remember, strong and shapely muscles are one of your best insurance policies against regaining fat.

The primary difference between muscle-maintenance and muscle-building routines is that you do not need to do as many exercises in maintenance. You've been doing a maximum of one set of ten exercises three times per week. You'll be able to reduce your number of exercises from ten to eight.

TRISH WHITE, AGE 24

"I CAN HARDLY BELIEVE IT—MY PANTS SIZE HAS GONE FROM A 14 TO A 5!"

Lost 25½ pounds of fat and trimmed 4 inches off her waist, 2¾ inches off her hips, 4¾ inches off her thighs in *twelve* weeks!

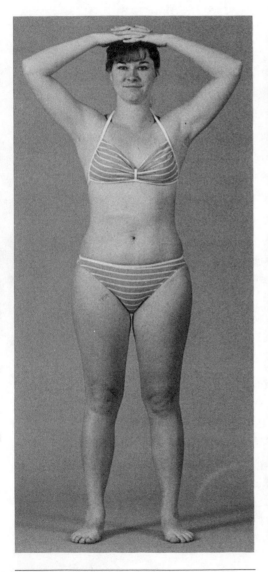

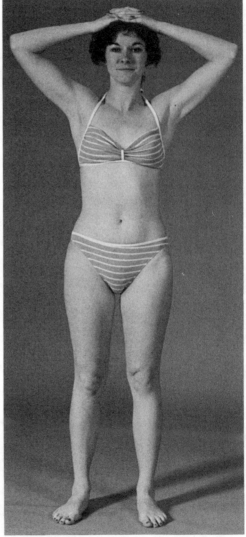

BEFORE
Six-Week Fat-to-Muscle Makeover.

AFTER
Six-Week Fat-to-Muscle Makeover.

Which exercises should you eliminate? It really doesn't matter, since the idea is to do slightly less exercise. In fact it's best to subtract a different two exercises with each new two-week period, adding the two you left out previously back to your routine.

Or you might want to experiment with new exercises. If so, I'll simply refer you to my 1988 revised edition of *The Nautilus Book.* Regardless of your routine, you should still adhere to the super-slow, high-intensity guidelines that you've been applying for the last several months.

Keep in mind that more exercise is not better exercise. Better exercise is harder exercise. Apply this concept consistently and the shape of your body may well exceed your goals.

14

■ANSWERING YOUR QUESTIONS ■

In any diet and exercise program there are always a multitude of topics that are covered only briefly. This opens the door to misunderstanding followed by questions, answers, and more questions. This chapter addresses many of those questions.

CHANGING FAT TO MUSCLE

Q ■ *The title of your book,* The Six-Week Fat-To-Muscle Makeover, *implies that you can turn fat into muscle. Can you actually change fat to muscle?*

A ■ No. Fat and muscle cells are as different as mayonnaise and marble. The chemistry of each simply won't allow you to change one to the other.

I chose to put "Fat-to-Muscle" in the title because it was more attention-getting than "Muscle-Fat" or "Fat-Muscle." It is common to refer to an overweight woman as "fat," when in fact she does have other components—such as muscle, bone, and organs—in her body. Likewise, a lean woman is said to be composed of "all muscle," which technically doesn't mean she is devoid of fat. She simply has a low percentage of body fat.

Both fat cells and muscle cells have the capacity to inflate or deflate. Like a balloon they can swell or shrink. The goal of *The Six-Week Fat-to-Muscle Makeover* is to increase the size of your muscle cells and decrease the size of your fat cells. And doing so requires proper exercise and proper diet.

DIETING LESS THAN SIX WEEKS

Q ▪ *I only want to lose approximately 7–8 pounds. How can I modify the six-week program to meet my goals?*

A ▪ You simply monitor your results at the end of each two-week period. If you're an average-sized woman, it should take you approximately four weeks to lose 7–8 pounds. At the end of four weeks, you then move directly into long-term maintenance—which is described in chapter 13.

Reaching her goals in four weeks is exactly what Ronda Hegar, a recent trainee of mine, did in Dallas, Texas, in the spring of 1988.

Ronda started the program weighing 120¾ pounds at a height of 5 foot 4¾ inches. With a body fat level of 22.3 percent, she already looked terrific in a bikini. But she wanted to look better.

Evaluating Ronda's before and after photographs on the following page proves that she made significant progress. In only

RONDA HEGAR, AGE 35

"FOR FOUR YEARS I RAN 35 MILES PER WEEK IN AN EFFORT TO REDUCE THE SIZE OF MY THIGHS. IT DIDN'T WORK. AFTER ONE MONTH OF THE MAKEOVER DIET AND EXERCISE PROGRAM, I REDUCED MY THIGHS NOTICEABLY."

Lost 10¼ pounds of fat and trimmed 1¼ inches off her waist, 1¼ inches off her hips, 2 inches off her thighs *in only four weeks!*

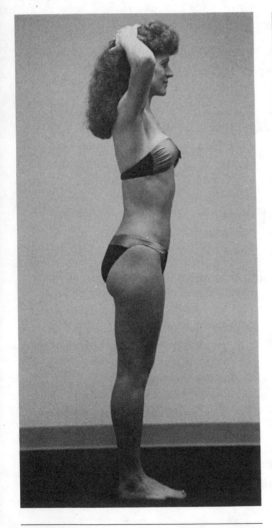

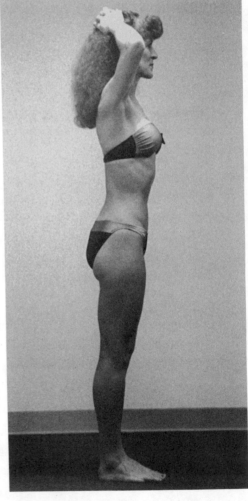

BEFORE
Six-Week Fat-to-Muscle Makeover

AFTER
Six-Week Fat-to-Muscle Makeover

four weeks she lost 10¼ pounds of fat and gained 2½ pounds of muscle. Her body fat came down to 14.6 percent. In addition, she removed 1¼ inches off her waist and 2 inches off her thighs.

"I used to jog five-to-six days per week, rarely leaving time to date," Ronda said with a slight smile on her face. "As a result of my improved figure, I now date five-to-six days per week, rarely leaving time to jog."

Ronda Hegar is a good example of what a woman with an attractive body can do in a short time to become even more attractive.

FAT-TO-MUSCLE MAKEOVER FOR MEN

Q ▪ *My husband has observed my dramatic fat loss on the Makeover program. Is it okay if he tries it?*

A ▪ The same general diet and exercise concepts apply to both men and women. The average overfat man, however, because he has significantly more muscle mass than the average overfat woman, requires more calories per day to keep his body healthy. Thus, placing the average overfat man on a daily diet of from 1,200 to 1,000 calories per day would not be safe in the long run.

I'd recommend that your husband start with 1,500 calories a day, and then gradually decrease his daily calories to 1,400, then 1,300. Men should never go below 1,300 calories per day. A specific fat-loss program for men is covered in detail in *The Nautilus Diet*.

REMOVING CELLULITE

Q ▪ *Will the Fat-to-Muscle Makeover remove cellulite?*

A ▪ Cellulite is just plain fat that accumulates in thick layers under the skin on the thighs and buttocks of women. It has a dimpled appearance, probably due to a honeycomb-like arrangement of the connective tissue and fat deposits in that area.

You apply the same strategy for eliminating cellulite as you do for removing fat anywhere else on your body. Unfortunately, the thighs and buttocks are generally an area of high fat concentration for women. It may be the first place fat accumulates on your body, and the last place it leaves.

The Makeover program's double whammy of building muscle to burn fat is the best course of action to take in combating cellulite—in lieu of the numerous bogus cures that are available.

EFFECT ON CHEST MEASUREMENT

Q ■ *Whenever I've lost weight, it's always seemed to come from my breasts. Will the muscle-building effect of the Makeover program stop that from happening this time?*

A ■ The lucky women of the world—at least in today's American culture—are those who store fat first in their breasts. But the opposite seems to be true for the majority—the initial dose of fat loss seems to come directly from the breasts.

Breasts are composed primarily of fat. Reducing fat means that your breasts will probably become smaller.

However, strengthening the muscle layer beneath the breast will add shape and contour. It will do a great deal to add firmness, combating the common problem of breasts sagging as you become older.

REST PERMITS GROWTH

Q ■ *Since the Fat-to-Muscle Makeover workouts are scheduled on alternate days, can I get better results by jogging or taking an aerobics class in between workouts?*

DEBBY WILLIAMS, AGE 35

"I BECAME EXCITED AS I STARTED SEEING THE WEIGHT COME OFF AND NOTICING MYSELF GETTING INTO BETTER SHAPE. I FELT LIKE I WAS ON A ROLL, ESPECIALLY DURING THE SECOND SIX WEEKS."

Lost 28½ pounds of fat and trimmed 3½ inches off her waist, 4¾ inches off her hips, 7¾ inches off her thighs in *twelve* weeks!

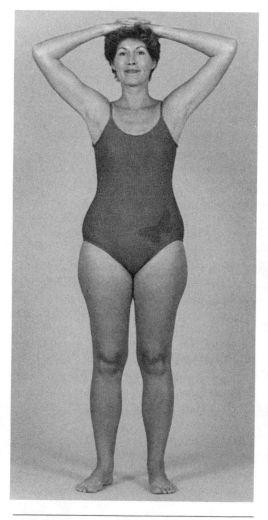 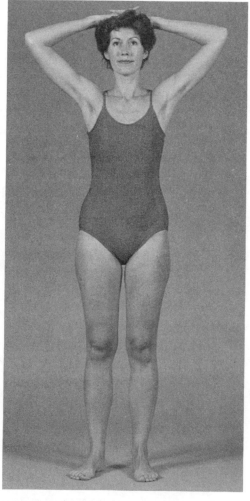

BEFORE
Six-Week Fat-to-Muscle Makeover.

AFTER
Six-Week Fat-to-Muscle Makeover.

A ■ No. You won't get better results, you'll probably limit your results. Don't forget that the goal of the program is to *build muscle* to burn fat. You may burn 150 calories by jogging, but you'll be stunting the progress you should be making in adding several pounds of figure-shaping muscle. An additional 4 pounds of muscle will burn an extra 200 to 400 calories each day, even at rest. Allow your muscles time to overcompensate and recover from the stress you placed on them. Then they'll grow stronger, bigger, more shapely—and burn more fat.

PLATEAU BUSTERS

Q ■ *When I seem to be stuck at a certain body weight, is there anything special I can do to start losing again?*

A ■ Plateaus will definitely test your patience, and your confidence in the program. We saw plateaus of various durations with the majority of women involved in the Fat-to-Muscle Makeover research projects.

Plateaus are natural; they are an inevitable part of successful fat loss. Here are some effective tips, however, that may shorten the length of your plateau.

- Drink lots of water. Water often acts as a stimulus. Have a glassful 10 minutes before every meal, and more during it. Be sure to drink plenty of water before, during, and after your workouts.

- Review your dietary calories. You may discover that a few extra calories have been slipping between your lips. Be honest with yourself and correct the situation.

- Make sure your workouts are high intensity and super slow. Effective workouts will add muscle to burn calories. Do not quit just because your muscles begin to burn. Push through the burn. By doing so, you'll stimulate the involved muscle to grow—and the next burn you feel will be fat leaving your body!

BROWN RICE PREFERRED

Q ▪ *Is it okay to use white rice instead of brown rice?*

A ▪ Brown rice is nutritionally superior to white rice. Because the nutrients in white rice are applied to the outside of the grain, they can easily be lost by rinsing or using too much water in the cooking process. It may be more difficult to find brown rice at the supermarket, but it is worth the effort to search.

TUMMY TRIMMER

Q ▪ *What specific exercises will flatten my stomach?*

A ▪ Both the Nautilus pullover and abdominal machines will *strengthen* your abdominal muscles. But your question implies a belief in spot reduction. There is no such thing. A fat-ordering process is programmed into your genes, and it dictates the location of your fat stores. Increasing your muscle mass throughout the entire body helps burn more calories, and will deplete those fat stores. But nothing can be done to pinpoint the area of reduction. Avoid the temptation to overdo abdominal exercises, since it could stunt your progress instead of helping it.

WHERE'S THE EGG?

Q ▪ *Until the optional Sunday brunch during the last two weeks, there are no eggs on this diet. Why?*

A ▪ Two or three eggs per week—within the calorie allotment— would be acceptable. However, the strategy of a daily Basic Breakfast necessitates leaving eggs off the menu. A daily egg would provide too much cholesterol.

KEEP VARIETY IN DINNERS

Q ■ *May I switch one dinner for another dinner; eating one twice during the week?*

A ■ It is best not to. A certain amount of variety is necessary. Optional alternate dinners are provided at the start of the third and fifth weeks.

HANDLING DINNER INVITATIONS

Q ■ *What should I do when I am invited to a friend's house for dinner?*

A ■ Explain that you are undergoing a Fat-to-Muscle Makeover. If an acceptable dinner can be arranged, fine. If not, and you do not wish to turn down the invitation, eat your evening meal in advance and join the party right after dinner.

RESTAURANTS AND FROZEN DINNERS

Q ■ *What restaurant foods would qualify for the diet, or how about commercially available frozen dinners?*

A ■ You are in treacherous territory. It is not impossible to achieve an acceptable meal through either means, but it is very difficult. McDonald's offers a Chicken Oriental salad that comes close to your Basic Lunch #2 Chef Salad, but bring your own dressing. Fish, broiled dry (no butter or fatty oils), a small salad (bring own dressing or use lemon and vinegar), and a plain baked potato would be an acceptable dinner. All in all, however, fast foods and most restaurant items have been prepared in oil, butter, or grease that adds excess calories.

As for frozen dinners, the chief culprit is sodium content. But if you can find a dinner with less than 850 milligrams of sodium, and less than 400 calories with about 50 grams of carbohydrate, 14 grams of fat and 20 grams of protein, enjoy it occasionally.

DOESN'T LIKE GARLIC

Q ▪ *Garlic is used in many of the evening meals. Since I do not like the taste of garlic, can I leave it out?*

A ▪ Yes, leave out the garlic. It will have no significant effect on the nutrient composition of the various meals.

GAINING MUSCLE

Q ▪ *Besides Lysa Parker, who is featured in Chapter 1, have you worked with any other woman who needed to gain muscle more than she needed to lose fat?*

A ▪ Yes. I recently trained Brenda Smedley, an engineer on our Nautilus staff in Dallas. Brenda, a dance enthusiast, stood 5 foot 5 inches and weighed 107 pounds. Her body fat was 16.4 percent, which was almost ideal. But her upper body was disproportionately weak (compared to her lower body) and needed more muscle. I convinced Brenda to let me put her on a Nautilus exercise program similar to the one in this book.

Since Brenda wanted to gain muscle more than lose fat, I recommended that she consume 2,000 calories a day. These 2,000 calories were derived by doubling the daily guidelines for 1,000 calories that are listed on page 48.

Brenda followed the exercise and diet plan faithfully. In six weeks, her body weight increased from 107 to 110¾ pounds. Her body fat decreased from 16.4 to 14.6 percent. And her strength improved approximately 50 percent in all her upper-body exercises. As a result Brenda lost 1.38 pounds of fat and added 5.13 pounds of muscle to her body. She also gained 2½ inches on her chest measurement.

Brenda proved, once again, that with proper exercise and proper diet a woman can take charge of the way she wants her body to look. In six weeks, or only eighteen high-intensity workouts, Brenda significantly improved her upper body and made her figure more symmetrical.

USING DUMBBELLS

Q ■ *I'm interested in performing the exercise portion of the Fat-to-Muscle Makeover with dumbbells. Did any of the women pictured in the book exercise with dumbbells, as opposed to using Nautilus?*

A ■ Yes. Sybil King, who is featured in Chapter 1, followed the recommended dumbbell routines. And as you can see, she received terrific results. The body-shaping benefits from proper exercise, as I stated in Chapter 12, are not so much in the equipment—but in *how you use* what you have available to you.

・ CONCLUSION ・

This diet and exercise program is for a woman who is serious about losing fat and keeping it off. It is for a woman who realizes that there are no quick and easy ways to reshape her body. And it is for a woman who enjoys the challenge of a disciplined diet and demanding exercise.

In short, the Six-Week Fat-to-Muscle Makeover is the most efficient way to thin thighs, slim hips, a flat stomach, and a simply stunning body!